NOT ANOTHER FITNESS BOOK

A Memoir ~ A Manual
A Message for 49 Million Baby Boomers

STEVEN HEAD, CSCS

ISBN: 978-1-7291-7190-5

*In loving memory of J. Rochelle "Shelly" Malone
& my little brother, Brian Andrew Head
I cannot go back, I can only go forward.
You both forgave me the moment you left.
At long last I have done the same.
I will live and love my life
Knowing now, all along, it's what you wanted me to do.*

CONTENTS

FOREWORD

I'VE WATCHED STEVEN Head transform his own life over nearly six years now.

Firsthand.

Which is why I feel both qualified and honored to write these words to you on his behalf.

This man "gets it." He gets it where others don't.

He understands fitness and the journey of mindset development like very few I have ever met in my life.

Right now, you may be in a hole. And you can see the crystal "blue skies" above you, but have no earthly idea how to get yourself out of this dark, suffocating place.

STEVEN HEAD

Maybe you've called up to the "marketer" or "guru" or "expert" walking by your hole in a plea for help.

But, as you likely now know, their advice and guidance is a mile wide but an inch thin.

Steven isn't going to offer you veiled advice.

He's going to jump down in the hole with you.

Because he's been where you are before.

And he knows the way out.

Give him a chance to help to you.

Because he can.

And he will.

Sincerely,

Brian Grasso
Mont Tremblant, Quebec
March 18, 2018

###

INTRODUCTION

"Give sorrow words; the grief that does not speak
Whispers the o'er-fraught heart and bids it break."

—William Shakespeare, *Macbeth*

THERE'S A STATISTIC kickin' around somewhere that suggests some eighty percent of Americans say they want to write a book, while only about one percent actually do it. Now I know why. That said, I am thrilled to have done so. And I'm thrilled you've decided to read it.

Thank you.

A caveat for the reader: there is both the memoir and the manual parts of this book, but each has elements of the other. I chose the title for good reason.

There are several quotes throughout this book. I encourage you to spend a little time reflecting on them. I invite you to ruminate on their message, the wisdom and insight contained therein.

This is, as you'll discover, a deeply personal book. Waking up to just how late in the game it truly is, I didn't hold much back. As cathartic and healing as this work has proven to be for me, the book's greater mission is to touch lives, to encourage, and to inspire. It also serves as my declaration to quit playing small and is an invitation for you to do the same.

My story, the memoir, might resonate with most anyone, particularly those who've battled depression or addiction or who have known profound, personal tragedy.

Throughout this project, I've had a few voices in my head. There was my own "Voice of Judgment" (aka the inner critic), and there were the judging voices I imagined from the fitness industry. But this book wasn't written for the fitness professional, even though I do hope many will read it. The manual part, the exercise information, was written for the *fitness disenfranchised*, for my fellow boomers who, for various reasons, are not living a fit, active lifestyle or who are floundering in their efforts to do so.

"Imagination is more important than knowledge. For knowledge is limited, whereas imagination embraces the entire world, stimulating progress, giving birth to evolution."

—Albert Einstein

One doesn't need to be an Einstein to realize imagination is ultimately more important than knowledge. Unless folks can imagine themselves succeeding, unless they can imagine themselves getting stronger and healthier, then all the knowledge in the world doesn't mean shit.

A number of years back, sitting in my home office on my yoga mat and looking across the room at my bookshelf, I remember suddenly being filled with a deep sense of gratitude for all the authors represented there. A couple decades' worth of reading—books that kept me company, that educated and inspired me; books that sustained me and gave me hope.

I can also recall thinking more than once how I admired anyone smart enough and knowledgeable enough about any topic to be able to write a book on it.

I didn't think I was. Didn't think I could.

Fast-forward that same number of years and what do ya' know. Between my life (on which I'm the world's leading expert) and my career in fitness, it seems I am, and, at long last, I have.

###

STEVEN HEAD

PART 1

My Life: Lost and Found

###

STEVEN HEAD

A "HOW-TO-THINK-ABOUT" BOOK

"The only true currency in this bankrupt world is the truth we share with one another when we are being uncool."

—Line from the movie, *Almost Famous*

"Other people are going to find healing in your wounds. Your greatest life messages and your most effective ministry will come out of your deepest hurts."

—Rick Warren

THIS IS MY hope. I'm not gonna lie: the thought of putting my life on paper, in a book, freaks me out. But it's something I felt I had to do. It felt like a much bigger risk *not* to. I did not want to add it to an already long list of regrets.

This book represents the facing of my fears head on, in the interest of healing for both reader and writer. For longer than I care to admit (okay, about ten years), I have been collecting notes and writing down ideas for a book I'd hoped to write someday. On May 2 last year, I sat down on my meditation cushion, opened my daily devotion book, *Offerings: Buddhist Wisdom for Every Day,* and read the quote for the day: "The trouble is, you think you have time."

It got my attention. I mean *really* got my attention.

I began to write.

So many of us live, for much of our lives, as though we will live forever, as though we have all the time in the world, without any sense of urgency, without any daily appreciation for how precious and unpredictable life is. I know I've been guilty of it.

Fear of failure, fear of scrutiny, a damaged self-image, a mindset at odds with prosperity, fear of public speaking—my personal demons—they've all caused me to put off writing a book. They convinced me to give up on dreams, to settle, to become way too comfortable with mediocrity. Ten years ago, however, a memoir in which I reveal my struggles, my heartbreaks, and my failures was *not what I had in mind.*

Time and circumstances have changed that.

I've seen how vicious the fitness industry's social media crowd can be. There is constant infighting on the Internet. It's an industry with more than its share of outsized egos, which often mask immense insecurities. The decision to make my life an open book *and* to offer up an unconventional, unapologetically non-scientific (as distinguished from unscientific) take on fitness advice was not an easy one.

An estimated forty-nine million baby boomers (those born between 1946 and 1964) are sedentary (around sixty-five percent of us). Forty-nine million who don't know the joy of movement, who don't realize the power of movement as medicine. This baby boomer thinks that's a tragedy. If I can reach even *forty-nine* of those people with this book and make a positive impact that I wouldn't have otherwise, then it will be worth any negative fallout.

"The greatest fear in the world is of the opinion of others, and the moment you are unafraid of the crowd you are no longer a sheep, you become a lion. A great roar arises in your heart, the roar of freedom."

—Osho

This is not another fitness book, but it is about a life in the fitness business. It's about the insights and the wisdom I've accumulated in a career that has spanned five decades in the fitness industry. (My first fitness job was in 1978.) I've come to realize and finally accept that I am very good at what I do, and what I have to share can be beneficial to almost anyone who has not yet succeeded, despite their efforts, to become fit and to make exercise a permanent part of their life, in order to reap the tremendous rewards of doing so.

Throughout my career, I've paid close attention to the more common stumbling blocks that trip folks up. The industry itself is complicit in a number of them. A great deal of confusion has been created by misinformation and conflicting views. A paralysis can set in when trying to make sense of it all. Hell, it's no wonder many of us can't find success in our fitness pursuit. I hope to help you with that.

Now, having said that, the biggest stumbling blocks are mostly a result of what goes on between the ears—attitudes that don't serve our best interests, misconceptions that hold us back, and limiting beliefs that we aren't even conscious to.

My own life experiences may be very different from yours. I have never been particularly out of shape. I've never been overweight. But those circumstances are merely symptoms of "challenges" we may very well have in common. I've suffered much of my adult life with issues of self-worth; I have had clinical depression that lasted for decades. I've struggled financially and had to declare bankruptcy, battled addictions (yes, more than one), and I have known personal tragedy that I used to joke with a counselor "would've killed a weaker man." My point is, *whatever* your fitness challenges—I mean your *deepest core challenges*—chances are I can relate to them.

"It's amazing how many people struggle with depression, anxiety and low self-esteem."

—A friend on Facebook

"The mass of men lead lives of quiet desperation, and go to the grave with the song still in them."

—*Walden,* Henry David Thoreau

So, no, this is not another fitness book, certainly not in the way one might ordinarily think of one. It is not a "how-to." It's not full of photos of attractive, enviable figures and physiques demonstrating a catalog of exercises.

Fitness how-to books number in the hundreds. Folks much smarter than I have written many of them. I'm fortunate enough to know a few of the awesome author-coaches who have written some of the best books out there. Theirs are among the books I've learned so much from and that have been key to my professional growth. Hundreds more run-of-the-mill fitness books are hanging out at the local bookstore. You may have one or two or twelve on your bookshelf now. Did they work? Did you learn an approach that resulted in a commitment to regular exercise? Chances are you did not. These books typically work best for those with a certain affinity and degree of self-motivation that many of us don't have. This is less about the Xs and Os, and more about the whys.

It is a "how-to-*think*" about exercise book. I will share my journey, my backstory, in the hopes of inspiring you to craft your own fitness philosophy, one that will sustain you and keep you committed the rest of your life. I will be "uncool" and share my "truth," vulnerable and unvarnished. I want to connect. One of my motivations is clearly catharsis, to exorcise some demons. To "write" some wrongs, if you will.

As a manual, I discuss here some practical aspects of training. Much of what I cover in this book might seem so basic that it scarcely warrants mentioning, and that might be true *were it not for the fact* that I encounter evidence to the contrary every day I spend on the fitness floor. I'm confident that a 4,000-member club in a major metropolitan market serves as a fairly representative microcosm of what goes on in clubs and gyms across the country.

I have been privy to some remarkable transformations along the way. If you knew just how powerful a mindful, simple, and sound approach to conditioning the body could be, if you had been witness to these transformations, you would understand my passion.

It is my fervent desire to help you become/stay active, engaged in life, and physically independent, and to help you avoid becoming yet another regrettable health-care statistic, at the mercy of a system that too often does not have your best interests at heart. In life, our health at times can seem like a crap shoot, but let's at least load the dice in our favor, shall we?

###

"You know what, Les? Sometimes we don't pick the books we read, they pick us."

That's a line from the movie, *Hurricane,* about boxing champion Rubin Carter, who is falsely accused and imprisoned for murder. While in prison, Carter writes a book, a copy of which ends up on a bargain table for twenty-five cents, from where the book "picks" a young boy whose parents end up helping Hurricane gain his release from prison. I was watching the movie one night on cable, and when I heard that line, I almost fell off the couch! It's a notion I have believed, thought, and voiced countless times over the years.

After graduating high school, I began to wake up from the *Fast Times* fog that characterized my high school daze.

The seeds for this [first stage of] awakening were an unlikely combination of scripture and television. My father was a religious man, but, more importantly, he was a spiritual man, meaning his faith was real. It was genuine, and it manifested in his wisdom, his compassion, and what he valued. For my high school graduation, I didn't get a car. I got a bicycle. My father also gave me a collection of some ten to fifteen books he thought would be of real value to a young man. One, of course, was a Bible.

The television I refer to was the show *Kung Fu* and specifically the lead role of Kwai Chang Caine. I was completely intrigued by the character's control of his emotions, his mental discipline, his calm, his equanimity. I saw a parallel in how the Gospels described Jesus.

The first time I felt as though a book *picked me* was in 1976. I was between high school graduation and my enlistment in the United States Air Force. Though I didn't yet know it as such, I was beginning to live an "examined life."

I walked into a bookstore, having no specific book in mind and only a vague notion of a subject. The book I stumbled upon was *Handbook to Higher Consciousness* by Ken Keyes, Jr. Its subtitle is *The Science of Happiness*. It was full of insight into how our thoughts and emotions create, limit, and distort our view of the world and of ourselves, if we remain *unaware* of their influence.

Mindfulness. It may seem trite, perhaps. *So easy to dismiss.* Yet nothing is more essential, nothing is more powerful, when it's ***understood*** and ***practiced***. What I learned from that book became a foundation for my work as a personal trainer/conditioning coach. I still have it; it sits on my bookshelf at home.

So, like Les in that bookstore, it is in this spirit of fate, providence, synchronicity—however you choose to think about it—that I offer this book. Perhaps this book finds you on the eve of starting an exercise program or on an exercise "hiatus." Or maybe you're about to give up on this "whole exercise thing," because results have proven elusive or because you keep getting injured.

You may be a relative newcomer to exercise or a seasoned veteran. You may think you know all there is to know about training, or you may know that you know very little. You may be absolutely flustered by all the experts and the information overload, not sure what to believe or who to trust.

Wherever you are in your "pursuit of fitness," chances are this book can be of value. It is aimed at those of "my g-g-generation." My contemporaries, baby boomers, stand to benefit the most and for whom it is most urgent. We have less time to squander. This demographic seems to be the least informed and most misinformed. In my experience, it is also the group of people most limited by fear.

STEVEN HEAD

"Many of our fears are tissue-paper thin, and a single courageous step would carry us clear through them."

—Brendan Francis

At our age, it's not about looking good naked so much anymore (not that there's anything wrong with that) as it is about forestalling an almost certain and precipitous decline into debility. It's about reversing the ill effects of decades of being deskbound, of having attended to life while neglecting our bodies.

Many of the health benefits come just from going from doing nothing to doing something. When we find the will and the why to overcome inertia, momentum can keep us in motion.

Behavioral psychologists suggest health as a focus is too abstract to be effective in motivating and sustaining change. That may very well be true when we are young and able-bodied. At thirty, it's hard to envision joint replacement, chronic pain, loss of mobility, or loss of independence. But, as the years accumulate, that abstract becomes more and more real. That's one reason I offer my story, in the hopes of helping you find something that resonates more deeply, something even more intrinsic, to ignite *your* passion, to stir *your* soul...

###

STEVEN HEAD

A MEMOIR: THE BEGINNINGS

MY FAMILY SETTLED into Fairfax City, Virginia, a suburb of Washington, D.C., in 1963. My father, a colonel in the U.S. Air Force, had been assigned to work at the Pentagon after the previous two years in Buenos Aires.

I was six years old. In short order, I met and made friends with about a half dozen kids up and down the street, all of us about the same age.

As far as we knew, there were only three sports that existed: baseball, football, and basketball. Most of us played all three. As the seasons changed, so did our game: Little League baseball, Fairfax Police Youth Club football, and basketball. We also played sandlot/pick-up games of each: baseball and football on what was known as the hockey field, where the Fairfax High School girls' field hockey team played; basketball in the driveway, a hoop and backboard mounted atop the garage.

I am so grateful I grew up before there were cell phones, video games, and computers. When we weren't playing organized or sandlot sports, we played tag, hide-n-go-seek, British bulldog, kick the can, badminton, and croquet. We also played pickle, a game that simulates a steal attempt and rundown of a base runner; and 500, a game where one got points for catching ground balls, line drives, and fly balls. We rode our bikes all over the place.

Physical activity was just a natural part of being a kid. But as we got older, started driving, and discovered girls, physical activity dropped off quite a bit. But part of the early '70s zeitgeist was a "return to nature," and backpacking became quite popular. Colin Fletcher's *The Complete Walker,* published in 1968, essentially launched the industry. A number of us read the book, caught the bug, and took up backpacking. By the time I went on my first hike, I was sixteen and had already been smoking cigarettes for a few years. The only exercise I was getting at that point was playing baseball.

If you've read Bill Bryson's *A Walk in the Woods*, then you might know where I'm going with this. Three or four of us drove down to the Shenandoah Mountains to hike up Mount Robertson. As mountains go, it barely qualifies, a mere 3296 feet, though it does have a fairly steep trail up to its summit. I just about died! With a pack weighing about thirty-five pounds for a weekend hike, it was the most physically demanding thing I'd done in my sixteen years.

This was a life-altering experience. An epiphany. A wake-up call. A number of things occurred to me on that hike. First, smoking and hiking don't mix very well. *Duh.*

Also, the absence of regular exercise left me woefully unprepared for the demands of backpacking, even at the tender age of sixteen. I had been taking my fitness, my health, for granted.

But the biggest impression I was left with, and one that inspired me to make a promise to myself that I've kept to this day, was the transcendent potential of... a walk in the woods. I realized how beautiful the mountains were, how peaceful it was, how... *therapeutic* being in the mountains could be. I knew I would want to do it again and again.

Though it would be two more years before I would kick my nicotine habit (for the first time), I vowed to get my ass in shape and keep it in shape, sufficient to be able to hike whenever the opportunity arose and so I could enjoy it, rather than suffer like I did on that first hike.

As a side note, a handful of my childhood friends have never given up backpacking. Some combination of us has made an annual *winter* hike for over forty years now.

###

A BROTHER. A FRIEND. A MOVIE STAR.

BURT REYNOLDS AND my older brother, Jeff, were two of the early inspirations who prompted me to take up weight lifting. Lewis Medlock, Reynolds's macho character in the 1972 film, *Deliverance*, stood in stark contrast to the spindly (or portly, in Ned Beatty's case), hapless city-slicker colleagues who accompanied him on that ill-fated canoe trip down the Cahulawassee River. Burt's/Lewis's "guns" were out of their holsters the entire movie, proudly, prominently displayed in his sleeveless wetsuit top.

I wanted to be Burt Reynolds.

At some point in high school, my brother began pumping some iron or, more accurately, sand-filled, plastic-coated weights from Sears & Roebuck. His biceps grew and I thought they looked awesome. I wanted to emulate a brother I had revered for much of my childhood, so I talked my parents into buying me a bench and a set of those sand-filled, plastic-coated weights.

You never forget your first pump.

This next story is a powerful one for me, profound and personal on a number of levels. Do me a favor and Google Ralph Hoar. (Read the *New York Times* obituary.) I'll wait...

Most people don't know who he was, yet millions owe him a debt of gratitude. I met Ralph when I was sixteen. He and his wife, Patsy, and their two kids,

Adrienne and Jason, moved into our neighborhood. He was twenty-eight.

He would turn out to be one of *the* most influential people to ever enter my life.

"Men are born soft and supple;
Dead, they are stiff and hard.
Plants are born tender and pliant;
Dead, they are brittle and dry.
Thus whoever is stiff and inflexible
Is a disciple of death.
Whoever is soft and yielding
Is a disciple of life.
The hard and the stiff will be broken.
The soft and supple will prevail.
　　　　　　—Lao-Tzu, *Tao Te Ching,* Chapter 76

I had put on a little muscle, pumping my sand-filled weights. Ralph occasionally hired some of the neighborhood kids to do work for him, like mow the lawn, paint. On one such occasion, I had done some painting of his fence. He invited me in during a break for tea or lemonade—can't remember. But what I do remember like it was yesterday was what transpired in his kitchen that day.

Ralph said to me, "It looks like you're pretty strong, but how flexible are you?"

With no sense at all about my flexibility, I just said I didn't know but assumed I was. Hell, I was sixteen. Why wouldn't I be flexible?

"Think you can do this?" He proceeded to get on the floor and roll up onto his shoulders with his legs rising up above his head. Then he let his legs drop back down, over, and behind his head, until his toes landed on the floor.

I figured I should be able to do that no problem. I got my legs up vertical as I perched on my upper back and shoulders. So far so good. But as I began to let my legs drop, my hamstrings, mid- and lower-back were having none of it! *WTF*? Tight! (No, I probably didn't really say or think "*WTF*"; the phrase hadn't been invented yet.)

When you're sixteen, someone twenty-eight, married, with two kids is *old.* And here was this "old guy" demonstrating flexibility I couldn't begin to approach. I asked him how that could be, how he achieved his flexibility.

"Yoga." was his answer. He had performed Halasana, aka plow pose.

I had not.

This was another epiphany, a big one. I thought to myself how is it someone that much older could be more flexible than me? At sixteen, I didn't know anything about the science of flexibility, nothing about the numerous factors that influence it. So, what I reasoned was, as people get older, most lose flexibility, but it was *not* the inevitable result of the passage of time. Rather, it was something we had control over, a result of either attending to and preserving, or neglecting it and losing.

Perhaps a bit simplistic, naïve even, but it served me well. I would later (three decades later) coin the phrase and refer to this phenomenon in a *Washington Post* article (written by my friend, Dallas Hudgens, who you'll meet later) as *premature rigor mortis.* I often say we are quite literally being robbed of life as we grow stiffer and stiffer. Think about it: what's a slang term for a corpse? A stiff!

A quick caution about yoga. It can mean any number of things to folks, depending on their experience or perception. Bad experiences and misconceptions, not to mention unqualified instructors, abound.

I went out the next day and bought a yoga book, *Yoga For All Ages* by Rachel Carr. I still have this one on my bookshelf. With the help of the book, I started and kept up a yoga practice for about eleven years before abandoning it. I resumed my practice while in massage therapy school, some ten years later, in 1996.

In addition to introducing me to yoga, which had a profound impact on me, Ralph introduced me to personal growth/consciousness-raising workshops that were big in the '80s and '90s. We attended a couple of them together. He was also a personal training client for a while. While I attended Marymount University, he had an apartment just a few miles away. We hung out and played countless hours of Trivial Pursuit, so much so that the same questions began popping up.

Ralph and I would remain close friends until his death in September of 2001. He was 56.

###

LIFTING, RUNNING, & JACK LALANNE

WHILE IN THE AIR FORCE, I took up distance running, either inspired by the running I had to do in basic training or, more likely, in spite of it.

In the first two and a half years of my tour, I ran almost every day, typically six miles at a time, on trails that ran through the woods, up, over and down hills on the backside of McChord Air Force Base in Washington State. On the weekends, I would drive the eighteen miles from the base out to Point Defiance Park and run the hiking trails that wound through the park, up and down longer, steeper hills. As my endurance grew, running became a tremendous pleasure, and this was a beautiful place to run. Pine needle beds padded the trails that treated hikers and runners to incredible views out over the Puget Sound all the way across to the Olympic Mountains.

At the peak of my running, I could finish a ten-kilometer cross-country (i.e., hills, uneven terrain) run in about thirty-five minutes. I always ran alone; it was a meditative experience, a joy. I never ran for a T-shirt, a trophy, or a medal.

But when the Air Force base sponsored a 10k run on the very cross-country course I ran almost every day, I decided to enter. After all, I had home-field advantage. It would be fun, I thought.

I remember it so clearly. The gun sounded and we were off, about twenty or thirty of us. I pulled up and dropped out within the first few minutes. It seemed that competing in the activity that had been a celebration of solitude, a moving meditation, completely "bogued" my [runner's] high. It robbed my running experience of all its intrinsic joy.

I also took up tennis while in the service. Competing on the court suited me much better. I played regularly for the next twenty-plus years.

More on baseball later. For now, it was the sport I played and enjoyed the most growing up. However, an injury in my senior year killed any ideas I had of playing after high school. The injury taught me many lessons retrospectively, lessons I've applied with my clients. Just two years after that injury, I took up playing tennis.

Most folks my age know who Jack LaLanne was. I learned of him during my Air Force years. He was already in his sixties and performing feats of strength and fitness that boggled the mind. This is a man who inspired the likes of Steve Reeves and Arnold Schwarzenegger.

I also learned about his early years, how he suffered with health issues as a kid, and how he found "'religion," i.e., discovered diet and exercise as a teenager. He made a lifelong commitment to a healthy diet and regular, vigorous exercise. And, as a result, he went on to live a long life, a very long life, and enjoyed a level of fitness and vitality through his sixties, seventies, eighties, and even into nineties that most folks never enjoy.

I remember consciously taking note of how fragile, immobile, sickly, and slow moving the typical senior citizen was in contrast to Jack LaLanne. When I first learned of him, then on throughout the rest of his life, I believed, though he looked like the exception to the rule, he should *be the rule* and *not* the exception. He wasn't an outlier particularly; not a genetic freak. In my mind, he was an example of what the human body is capable of, how it is actually intended to function, if we only gave it proper care… and respect.

I get that LaLanne's workouts were long and his feats legendary, but I stand by my premise. Much more modest efforts will still yield remarkable results. He was fond of saying, "People don't die from old age. They die from inactivity." There's a lot of truth to that, and the worst part is so many of us suffer all manner of maladies, both systemic and orthopedic, long before we go. Long before many of us are old chronologically, we are old biologically!

At some point, in high school I quit weightlifting and I didn't pick it up again until after almost three years of running six to ten miles a day. Looking in the mirror one day, I thought, "Damn, I'm skinny!" Almost overnight, I retired my Nike running shoes and decided to take up bodybuilding.

Talk about two opposite ends of the spectrum! My practice of learning from the best began early on. Published in 1977, *Arnold: Education of a Bodybuilder* became my textbook.

Since my body weight had been reduced so much from all the running, my muscular development in the first year was rather dramatic. After thirteen months, I entered my first (and only) amateur bodybuilding competition, Mr. Tacoma. I placed third, got my photo in the local newspaper, and was quoted in the accompanying article.

That was the extent of my bodybuilding "career." I had no interest in pursuing it any further, realizing I lacked the genetic makeup to be seriously competitive, and I refused to even consider a bigger body through chemistry, i.e., no steroids for me, no thank you very much. Over the years, when discussing this transition from scrawny to muscular, and showing folks the before and after photos, I often got asked about whether or not I had any "help."

After my discharge from the service, I took up running again, yet continued a bodybuilding-type training routine.

I liked the balance.

As short-lived as each of my forays to opposite ends of the metabolic continuum were, they both proved invaluable in informing my work over the years, both with athletes and the "average Joes and Janes," who make up the majority of my clients.

These are some of the early influences and revelations that made big impressions on me. There would be many more. Collectively, they played a huge role in helping me decide what I wanted to be when I grew up. Yet, for all their influence, they hardly begin to explain why I stayed with this profession and have so much passion for it almost forty years later...

JOB INSECURITY

"If exercise could be packed into a pill, it would be the single most widely prescribed and beneficial medicine in the nation."

—National Institute of Aging

BETWEEN 1984 AND 1990, I worked in several places. I was a Nautilus instructor during my senior year in college. I worked briefly as a sales rep for a company that retailed exercise equipment, and designed and outfitted small amenity-type workout rooms for hotels and office parks. It was a mom-and-pop venture, and it went out of business.

STEVEN HEAD

I was the fitness director at a club in Fairfax, Virginia; it, too, went out of business. I got hired as a trainer by a mad-scientist-type and his business partner, who were opening a club that was going to feature some forty-plus pieces of Nautilus equipment, which the two of them were going to computerize to monitor reps and tempo. And, though I can't be sure, probably to administer an electric shock as well, if you tried to do more than one set.

The Nautilus Kool-Aid flowed freely. I just wanted a job. So, I drank. Eight of us were hired, and we worked for two months helping get the place ready to open. We opened before they ever got the computerization to work. Within a year, the partners still hadn't pulled it off and were at each other's throats. The grandiose venture went belly up as well. The club was called Neo-Med. I have to give them credit: as the name suggests, they saw the connection.

So, my track record of going to work for fledgling companies in the hopes of benefiting from being there on the ground floor was pretty bad. Career-wise, I was spinning my wheels.

After all that, in 1989, I went to work for a personal training center, probably the first of its kind in the area. I would actually do two stints with this company, The One To One Fitness Center. My first stay was pretty short, less than two years. I don't recall the decision to leave and not sure why I did, but I do know it wasn't because they went out of business! I came back to work for them from 1994 until 1998. The owner told me I was welcome to come and work for him whenever I wanted or needed. They are still going strong today. It was there I met a woman who would forever change my life; more on her a bit later.

In 1990, I saw a want ad for a physical therapy company looking to hire someone to perform fitness assessments on their patients. When I interviewed with the owner, I asked him what he had in mind for his patients *after* the assessment. He hadn't really thought about it, oddly enough.

But I had.

I did some research prior to my interview and found out this company had a number of physical therapy clinics in the area. I proposed he and I team up and open a personal training studio inside one of his clinics. To me, it was a perfectly logical arrangement.

I explained it to him this way. The average PT patient prior to injury is well to the left on the fitness/physical capacity continuum. Injury pushes them further to the left. Typical physical therapy treatment brings them back to the right, but not even back to pre-injury status. I argued strength training was the key to extending his patients' recovery, and personal training was a great way to enhance his services beyond the end of their therapy prescription. He agreed.

This concept, held by many in my industry as almost self-evident today, was anything but, twenty-nine years ago.

We equipped a small office down the hall from one of his clinics as a sort of a test run. We had a StairMaster, a PTS Turbo 1000 [true] recumbent bike, a Hoist-brand home gym, an adjustable bench, and a rack of dumbbells.

The position I essentially talked myself into required me to do one-on-one training full-time, which I had done for the previous two years, but only in a format where the clients weren't assigned to one specific trainer. At the One To One Fitness Center, clients rotated among trainers. Being the only trainer for everyone in a small space where it's just you and the client is a whole other animal. This approach really puts the "personal" in personal training. Be careful what you ask for, right?

For an insecure introvert, having to be "on" hour after hour, one-on-one actually freaked me out. I had my first anxiety attack the evening after he offered me the job. It was a relatively minor one.

###

FOUR FUNERALS AND A HEALING

"Mr. Duffy lived a short distance from his body."

—James Joyce

DEPRESSION AND LOW BACK PAIN: I've known both. Odds are you've known one or the other, as well. The statistics on back pain are staggering. One of my earliest clients in my newly created position was a fifty-five-year-old retired Navy man who came to me with both. I don't recall who referred him, but I will never forget our training and the outcome. I still have his testimonial letter.

He was sedentary; I suppose being "middle aged" and adjusting to life after the Navy weighed on his psyche. I knew almost nothing back then about movement patterns, corrective exercise, and the like, so it was just dumb luck and a testament to the power of exercise that we achieved such great results together.

Within a few months of our working together, both his depression and low back pain began to recede. His doctor took him off antidepressants. When he stopped training with me (about a year later), he spent roughly $40,000 building an addition onto his house, where he replicated the gym we began our training in. And yes, his name *was* Duffy. True story.

People who stick with a sound, consistent training approach usually report feeling "better," a notable outcome, if not somewhat nebulous. Relief from back pain *and* depression? Mr. Duffy got to feeling better in spades.

But the desire to *look* better was, and still is, a primary motive for many. I saw a lot of this early in my career. It's certainly why I took up bodybuilding. Early on, I lacked an appreciation for the connection between exercise and health. I did not understand exercise's potential to be a *powerful medicine.* For the most part, our culture still viewed exercise as a vain indulgence, not recognizing the connection either. In a similar vein, I often got reactions that reflected this perception when I answered the question, "What kind of work do you do?"

When I answered, common follow-ups were, "Is that your real job?" "Do you do that full-time?" "Is that all you do?" Sometimes the response was just, "Oh." They didn't need to say any more.

Powerful medicine, indeed. I would learn just *how* powerful in the coming years. By 1977, at age twenty, I had already lost three loved ones: a close childhood friend, Michael Rodio, when I was fifteen; my older sister, Glenda, when I was sixteen; and then a girl whom I'd met my senior year in high school and fallen in love with, named Holly Mobley.

I had known Michael since I was seven. We played sandlot ball, rode our bikes, built forts, and played pool in his garage. My sister was sixteen in 1964 and a *huge* Beatles fan. I was seven and lost out to her obsession on February 9, when, instead of watching *The Scarecrow* on Walt Disney's *Wonderful World of Color*, we had to turn the one and only TV to the *Ed Sullivan Show.* I became a Beatle fan that night, as well.

After graduating high school in 1966, Glenda went on to attend Mary Washington College. During her freshman year, she began to suffer constant, debilitating headaches. She was diagnosed with a brain tumor. They operated on her to remove it, but the surgery left her partially paralyzed, unable to walk. Her beautiful blonde hair never came back, and her speech was badly affected. She lived another seven years before passing away in June of 1973.

Holly and I took notice of each other my senior year in high school, though she was only a sophomore. We slowly became acquainted and developed a friendship. We hung out a few times after I graduated in 1975 and before shipping off to the Air Force in '76. We corresponded quite a bit during my basic training and during tech school, continuing even after I settled in Washington State at my permanent duty station.

Our friendship was morphing; I was falling in love. There are some things you just never forget, like your first kiss of a new romance, even if it's only in a dream. We had not been "romantic" yet; we hadn't had that first kiss. I was in bed asleep one morning in the barracks; the only phone was in the hallway where all the airmen took and made their calls. I got a loud knock on the door that woke me from a dream.

"Phone call for Airman Head!"

The call was my mother informing me of Holly's death. She'd been driving her little Chevette in a snowstorm between home and school at East Tennessee State University, lost control, and gone off the road.

The dream that my mom's call woke me from was of Holly and me kissing for the first time. In the days that followed, I walked around the base with James Taylor's "Fire and Rain" playing in my head. I always thought I would see her again.

Each loss, heartbreaking in itself, collectively took quite a toll. They left me vulnerable to depression, as would be explored in counseling many years later. That counseling, in 1992, lasted three months. Without health insurance, I couldn't afford it any longer. Three months is also how long my first and only prescription for antidepressants lasted. It ran out, and I never refilled it.

I entered into counseling (pastoral counseling: therapy on the cheap) after yet another painful loss. This time, it was the woman I was deeply in love with and had hoped to marry. Her name was Shelly Malone. She's the woman I met while working at the personal training center. You can Google her, as well. *Unsolved Mysteries. Washingtonian Magazine. Washington Post. Fauquier-Times Democrat. The Middleburg Mystique.*

After a yearlong romance then another year as close friends, we "re-consummated" our relationship. It was a late September Sunday. After we made love, I decided I would ask her to marry me on her birthday in December. This was following a horseback ride we took together along the trails around "Western View," her home in The Plains, Virginia. I rode the horse that, less than a month later, would be blamed for her death.

She was a complicated woman, as was our relationship. Her story is tragic. Her death absolutely devastated me, and I sank into a depression that would last for years.

In the years following Shelly's death, exercise became a lifeline. I have said many times I likely would not have made it without it. Each workout, with its dose of endorphins, gave me temporary relief from the otherwise relentless despair. Each time I willed myself to the gym, it was an exercise in hope, in self-determination. I am convinced exercise is as powerful an antidepressant as there is.

###

S.A.D.

THERE ARE A NUMBER of more costly, more destructive addictions than cigarette smoking, but for a fitness pro/personal trainer, being a smoker is plenty costly and plenty destructive. The toll is first and foremost, emotional.

I have had two long stretches where I smoked. The first started when I was about ten. I didn't smoke heavily. At that age, occasions to sneak a cigarette were few. Once I reached high school and certainly when I started driving, I began smoking more heavily and was, without a doubt, addicted. I smoked right up until two days before graduating high school. I quit cold turkey.

The second stretch began when I was in college and dating a smoker, someone I met while working as a doorman/bouncer at a restaurant. I began by mooching a few drags off hers and then an entire cigarette. In no time at all, I was addicted again. I was a closet smoker for roughly fourteen years during that go 'round. About half of that time, I barely smoked: five a day or less. The other half, I smoked close to a pack a day. During the day I might smoke one, maybe two cigarettes, but after work, at night, I could easily smoke close to a pack.

I was not living a lie, but it was far too easy for many to see it that way and to judge me as such. It seemed a lot of people took some degree of sadistic satisfaction (Can you say, "Schadenfreude?") in pointing out how hypocritical they thought it was. It wasn't hypocrisy; it was a paradox, a dichotomy. Keeping it a secret was an act of self-preservation. I was protecting my spirit, my psyche.

I never lectured anyone while I was a smoker myself, nor in the years after becoming a non-smoker. I never judged them. I was a closet smoker, but a smoker nonetheless. I could actually empathize with them; I understood their predicament. If one has never been addicted to cigarettes or anything else, it's almost impossible to appreciate what a powerful grip it can have and how powerless one can feel.

I was, in fact, far more fit than many of those who judged me for smoking. I was committed to regular exercise despite my addiction. There are actually studies showing those who smoke yet exercise have better health outcomes, including lower morbidity and mortality rates, than those who don't smoke but who are sedentary.

Nonetheless, living under the specter of scrutiny and fear of judgment can create a real sense of shame. Shame is a bitch. It can be incredibly destructive. Shame around sexual matters is probably the worst. "Toxic shame" is the term given to it by psychologists, therapists, and counselors. It's something so painful that even admitting it to oneself is often too much to handle. Shame is something one just doesn't talk about, doesn't admit to. Not until psychotherapy or until one decides to write a book, that is.

Shame. Addiction. Depression. The three feed off each other, creating a vicious, synergistic cycle. The acronym is apropos; I was indeed *sad*, desperately so, for a long, long time.

I had another epiphany while working for the physical therapy clinic. Two years in, I was not making a go of the personal training center. I was just struggling to survive, both emotionally and financially. I was on the verge of bankruptcy. In 1994, I declared bankruptcy.

My depression was so debilitating, so absolutely exhausting, I could not accomplish the work needed to grow the business. To make matters worse, spending money (money I didn't have, via credit cards) had become one of my coping strategies. The pressure never let up. The inability to pay my bills, my profound despair following Shelly's death, and the unrelenting stress: I became convinced there was a connection between all of it and the excruciating low-back pain I was suffering.

I tried to tell my boss (a physical therapist) there was connection between the emotional stress and my low-back pain. He scoffed, suggesting it had to be something I was doing in the gym, a lapse in technique or a poorly chosen exercise. I knew better.

There are highly regarded spine/back pain specialists that would beg to differ (I know this firsthand), asserting there is no connection between emotional pain/psychological stress and low-back pain. But suggesting someone's back pain is all in their head

[63]

and not "real" is very different from actual physical pain that has as its origins in one's response to psychological stress.

Dr. John Sarno's work and his Tension Myositis Syndrome theory are still "controversial" and not widely accepted throughout the medical community. Yet there *is* the more commonly accepted notion that stress causes many folks to unconsciously shrug and hold their trapezius and neck muscles tight and "guarded," resulting in chronic neck pain. I'm not sure why low-back pain should be any different, if someone guards and tenses in that area of the body in response to stress.

One's personal, firsthand experience of some things can cause a questioning of conventional wisdom. And it's remarkable how a long "dark night of the soul" can change one's perspective... on a number of things.

There was a massage therapist on staff at the time. I can't recall if she persuaded me to get on her table or if it was a decision I made on my own. I had had a massage or two in the late 1980s and was convinced it was a powerful tool, a healing art. I had even thought about going to massage school, but none of that prepared me for what would happen on her table that day.

In body worker circles, it's referred to as an "emotional release." As she worked on me, I could feel it "bubbling up." Try I as did, I couldn't quell it. I broke down. I began to sob. Reflecting on it later that night, I saw it as an example of how our bodies can be an archive of painful emotions, of unresolved "wounds." The decision to enroll in massage therapy school would come a few years later. It seemed like a perfectly natural skill set to complement my personal training.

###

Another event in 1994 had a huge impact on how I thought about my work. Snow. Lots of it. That alone seems inconsequential, but the news reported there were more than a dozen deaths associated with shoveling that snow. I surmised these people were, in all likelihood, sedentary; not in good shape. Instead of the shoveling being just another workout of sorts, it killed them.

My personal, firsthand experience with low-back pain didn't end there. A couple years later, I enrolled at the Potomac Massage Training Institute. And, once again, I found myself under extreme stress. Between tuition costs and working for a personal training company that didn't pay much, I struggled to keep my head above water.

This time, it was much worse. I remember a couple episodes that absolutely crippled me. My back went into complete spasms, resulting in a level of pain I'd never experienced before—from *anything* and, thankfully, never since. It was like being stabbed, or how I imagine being stabbed must feel, having never actually been stabbed.

I mentioned earlier how I had abandoned my regular yoga practice. In the midst of my excruciating pain, I began to rethink that move. Physical tightness, hyper-tonicity, an unconscious "guarding" in response to emotional/psychological stress, resulting in physical pain—that's how I saw it. At times, I would catch myself guarding, tensing in my low back and hips.

Yoga was originally a spiritual practice. It's primarily a meditative art. Yoga poses done without a meditative, mindful approach are nothing more than stretches or, as B.K.S. Iyengar once noted, "calisthenics with Sanskrit names." This distinction cannot be overstated!

Meditation in its simplest form is a conscious, deliberate directing of one's attention, typically to the breath. Breathing consciously usually results in a deeper, more efficient breath, which in turn elicits something known as the relaxation response.

"Relaxation response" is a term coined by Harvard M.D. Herbert Benson, the modern day father of mind-body medicine. He preferred relaxation response to meditation because he thought it was more "scientific." That's somewhat ironic when you consider that the words meditation and medicine share a very similar etymology. The relaxation response is essentially the physiological opposite of the stress response, aka. the fight-or-flight response. Most of us are far more familiar with that one.

I reasoned that yoga, when practiced as a meditation, could help reduce both the mental stress and the physical tightness it created. So, I resumed my practice. That was 1996. In the twenty-two years since, I have never suffered anything close to that kind of pain.

Correlation doesn't prove causation—I get that. It's impossible to know how big a role yoga played in avoiding any subsequent episodes. I've never been that strapped financially again, either. Many low-back-pain cases clear up on their own, eventually. Regardless, I was sure I'd rediscovered a practice that would make a great long-term strategy going forward. Stress is ultimately an "inside job"; it's created by our perceptions, our interpretations of circumstances and events.

It became clear to me that yoga and meditation (or just yoga *as* a meditation) could be powerful practices for emotional and physical health.

Another seminal book in both my personal and professional development was *Full Catastrophe Living* by Jon Kabat-Zinn, written in 1990. Its subtitle is *Using the Wisdom of Your Mind and Body to Face Stress, Pain and Illness.* I cannot begin to do justice to the impact this book had on me. It's the reason I decided to enroll in yoga teacher training. In 1979, Kabat-Zinn founded the Stress Reduction Clinic at the University of Massachusetts Medical Center. This book describes the program there, which is founded on yoga and mindfulness meditation. It continues to this day, almost forty years later.

###

DALLAS FROM ATLANTA

I MENTIONED DALLAS HUDGENS earlier. He wrote the *Washington Post* article on yoga I was interviewed for in 1998. The way I met him was pretty cool. It was 1991, my first year running the little personal training studio. I had set out one day with a bunch of brochures to canvass a nearby neighborhood of single-family homes. When I finished, I had three brochures left.

Right behind the medical building where I worked was a townhouse development of around sixty units. It was up and across from the houses I'd just hit. Heading back to the studio, I decided to walk down the long drive that ran through them. Standing literally in the middle of the road, surrounded by sixty front doors, my remaining three brochures in hand, I paused and waited for some inspiration. I'm not sure I really expected to receive any, but it was fun to pretend like I might. Moved by the spirit ... or not ... I picked the three. One of them turned out to be Dallas's. (I think I picked his house because there was a bike rack on top of his car; there ya go—inspiration enough!) His wife, Deborah called me the next day.

"We're born again, there's new grass on the field."
—John Fogarty, "Centerfield"

They both became clients and, soon thereafter, good friends.

We lost touch for a couple years (he moved back to Atlanta for a short while), and, unbeknownst to me, he started playing adult recreational baseball in 1995.

Dallas had been researching an article for the Weekend section of the *Post* on recreational baseball leagues in the D.C. area, and he ended up joining the team he wrote about: Team 6 of the Ponce De Leon Men's Baseball League.

You'd think, as significant as this day turned out to be, I'd remember it in more detail, but I don't. Sometime in late 1997, Dallas and I were hanging out, and he asked me if I played baseball. I assumed he meant as a kid.

I said something like, "Yeah, in a former life I did." I explained how I'd hurt my shoulder in high school during senior year and hadn't played since. He told me about the league he'd joined and how much fun it was.

We both knew my shoulder could handle the demands of tennis. Maybe it could also handle baseball. I hadn't really even thought about baseball much since 1975, let alone considered playing it, and had no idea there were adult leagues. I didn't even follow Major

League Baseball. Sure, in the '80s I'd heard about the "Wizard of Oz," Ozzie Smith, with the St. Louis Cardinals. It was hard to miss the buzz created by Cal Ripken, Jr., Sammy Sosa, and Mark McGuire in the mid-nineties. Beyond that? *Meh*. Sour grapes, I suppose.

But Dallas got me thinking. Surely my arm could handle a few throws per game to a cut-off man. I could play the outfield. Seven out of my ten years playing as kid, I either pitched or played shortstop. I had my doubts about returning to either, but outfield seemed doable.

In the spring of 1998, I joined Ponce De Leon Baseball Team 6 to play ball for the first time in twenty-three years, alongside my friend, whom I'd met because he had a bike rack on his car.

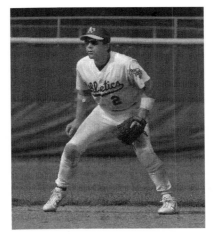

Head at shortstop

###

THE AGE AND AGEISM OF BASEBALL

"How old would you be if you didn't know how old you was?"

—Satchel Paige

MY RETURN TO BASEBALL was, forgive me, a real game changer. It got me to look at training in a whole new way. I realized my old bodybuilding approach wouldn't optimize my performance on the diamond.

I began to view my clients' training differently, as well. Athletes move. Bodybuilders pose. Maybe my clients would benefit more from training that looked more like sports conditioning than bodybuilding, unless of course the client actually wanted to body build.

In his book, *Ultimate Back Fitness & Performance,* Dr. Stuart McGill writes, "Bodybuilding principles specifically designed to hypertrophy muscles have become widespread in both rehabilitation and in performance training, yet they are often a detriment for achieving optimal health and athletic performance."

Another way returning to play at forty-two changed the game was the ageism I encountered.

A couple definitions of ageism:

1) The tendency to draw conclusions about an individual based on chronological age alone.

2) Negative attitudes towards the process of aging or toward older individuals.

It was a co-worker, of all people, who fired the first salvo. "Don't you think you're a little old to be playing baseball?"

I can't tell you how many times I got asked, when someone saw me in uniform, was I a coach? Or did I have a son who played? Or how many times, when I told someone I played baseball, they came back with, "Softball? You mean softball?" It seemed too much of a stretch for so many to imagine someone my age playing fast-pitch hardball. And it only got worse the older I got. In spring 2018, a few months shy of my sixty-first birthday, I take the field for my twenty-first season.

Ageism is an insidious and destructive force. Much of the physical decline associated with age is a self-fulfilling prophecy based on misinformation and poor role models, not to mention the continuous and concerted effort by pharmaceutical companies, through their relentless advertising, to convince us we are a bunch of hapless saps who need a laundry list of meds just to get through the day. It has far less to do with the passage of time and far more to do with failing to preserve strength and mobility.

Changing attitudes on aging became one of my missions. My performance, my success as an "old man playing a kid's game," reinforced my commitment to my work. It inspired me to take on prevailing attitudes, and it brought to life the truth, "We don't stop playing because we get old; we get old because we stop playing." At an age when most guys have since retired from their co-ed softball league, I was just getting started.

###

PANIC IN FALLS CHURCH

"I stand in awe of my body."

–Henry David Thoreau

"If anything is sacred the human body is sacred."

—Walt Whitman

BASEBALL OFFERED SOME respite, but I was still suffering. The devastated state Shelly's death left me in was not going away. Though it had eased some, it created a mass of collateral damage. No relationship, for example; I was "emotionally unavailable" as they say. More financial struggle. More isolation.

My father died in 1996, just as I was finishing up massage school. This left my mother, his wife of fifty-one years, alone in the house I grew up in. My father was so at peace throughout his life, a man of deep, authentic faith. Our relationship was solid—no unresolved issues. Losing him didn't have near the impact it might have had otherwise.

While the ostensible reason for my next move sounds altruistic, noble, it was really just a cover to minimize the shame and humiliation I felt around it. I moved back home, *at thirty-nine*. Let that sink in a minute.

I told folks it was to be there for my mother, to ease her loss, so she wouldn't feel so alone. There *was* that, sure. I was in a position to do it and knew it would be good for her. But the bigger truth was that it offered me much-needed relief from my financial hardship.

The night before the move back home, I had my second and most severe anxiety attack. This one scared the shit out of me. I had gone with a pool-shooting friend back to his house after closing down the pool hall. A beer or two and something to eat was the mission. It turned out a certain "medicinal herb" was also among the offerings. No doubt the partaking of said substance exacerbated the anxiousness I felt about moving back home and all its ramifications. My heart began to flutter and pound. I struggled to get air as my breath got increasingly ragged and shallow. I was freaking out.

I told my buddy, "We gotta call an ambulance! I'm fuckin' dying! We're gonna have to tell 'em what I did."

As you might imagine, he wasn't too keen on the idea.

He tried to calm me down. "Just relax. You'll be fine." Something like that. He persuaded me to lie down on the couch.

By then, I was in less of a panic, though far from okay. I lay on my side, head on a pillow, and I began to hear and feel my pulse. I became aware of my breath, and it was this biofeedback that enabled me to diffuse the attack. I had elicited the relaxation response. I had activated my parasympathetic nervous system.

###

I mentioned here earlier that I smoked. Some folks with less addictive tendencies can pick up cigarettes and put them down at any time. I was *not* one of those folks. You've probably heard it said nicotine is more addictive than heroin, harder to quit. I wouldn't know about that. All I know is quitting, particularly in the middle of a deep and chronic depression, was the hardest thing I've ever done.

STEVEN HEAD

My craving for a cigarette felt a lot like a small-scale anxiety attack. I fought my addiction for years but never made this connection. I smoked for almost fifteen years (the second round) and tried to quit for about ten of them. On every holiday and every other significant date that came along, I would try to quit. It wasn't until I consciously, consistently began to "sit" with every craving as it came up, turning my awareness to my breath, softening my belly, letting it rise and fall as I breathed, it wasn't until I rode my breath through and past the cravings that I succeeded in quitting. That's meditation in its simplest form. Powerful, *powerful* medicine.

Finally, on February 14, 1998, I did it. One day at a time.

###

BRIAN ANDREW HEAD

MY PARENTS HAD four children. I've mentioned my two older siblings. I also had a younger brother—*had*.

Brian was eight years younger than I. We had a very good relationship, though not especially close, given the age difference. In October 1999, on Columbus Day weekend, I was driving back from a get-together of my childhood friends at one of their cabins on the Shenandoah River. Driving down Route 211 on my way home, I was less than two miles from Brian's house at one point. I remember debating whether to pull off and go visit him. I decided against it and instead continued

[85]

on into Warrenton to shoot some pool at the local pool hall.

It's a decision I will regret the rest of my life. I never got another chance to see him. On October 31, my little brother took his life.

The guilt. The loss. The fucking pain. It was *almost* enough to make me to want to do likewise. Shelly's death almost ended me. At times, I thought losing Brian, especially this way, *actually would*. In 1999, I was just beginning to see light at the end of the tunnel following Shelly's death. You know what they say about that light at the end of the tunnel: sometimes it's a fucking train.

Losing a loved one to suicide—I'm not sure there's anything much worse. You wonder what you could have done, what did you miss, did you contribute to it somehow? The worst part, however, is realizing just how much pain they must have been in, how sad and hopeless they must've felt for so long.

During the years following Shelly's death, I had dreams in which I cried, I mean *CRIED*, from deep in the soul, a primal, guttural, full-body, convulsing wail. Up to this point, only in dreams, but in the shower on the morning following Brian's suicide, that prophetic nightmare came to life.

When faced with this kind of tragedy, loss, it seems we have one of two choices: we can let it make us bitter and mad at the world, perhaps resigned to a life of sadness, or we can look for grace.

"Though hard to bear, the sorrow and the shame, the anger, the fear and fatigue—each is a gift. For each can bring into focus our deep interconnection in the web of life. And lift us out of our narrow selves and bring us into community across space and time. Each can open us to the boundless heart. Though found in pain, that boundless heart is real, and the ground of all healing."

—Joanna Macy

In the weeks and months following, people I'd known for some time told me about how they'd lost a sibling to suicide. I'd had no idea. There is such a stigma around it. There's a sense of shame for those left behind—it's difficult to talk about. But what I began to become conscious to was how not uncommon it was, and how universal tragedy, suffering, and loss truly are. Compassion, for others and for *myself,* was the only choice.

"Get busy living or getting busy dying."
    —Andy Dufresne, *The Shawshank Redemption*

While the choice was easy enough, actually living it was anything but. Functional depression. Dysthymia. The current term/diagnosis is Persistent Depressive Disorder, when someone suffers from chronic, clinical depression but is able to function well enough to get through the day. But functioning at such a low level as I was really ain't living. It's a hell of a lot more like dying. Or sleepwalking. This is what it felt like for me, for more than twenty years.

###

RACKING UP DAMAGE. BREAKING BALLS. BANKING ON BRIAN.

"Your worst enemy cannot harm you as much as your own unguarded thoughts."

—Buddha

"Let's to billiards."

—William Shakespeare

I'VE DONE A FAIR amount of introspection and self-analysis through the years. There was the three months in actual counseling following Shelly's death. There were a few multi-day intensive personal growth workshops going all the way back to the mid-eighties, with Lifespring then Landmark Forum and Temenos, in the nineties. I've read probably close to a hundred books on related topics—personal growth, psycho-spirituality, and behavioral science. As powerful as it all was, as much as I learned, and as much as it contributed to the wisdom I possess today, it could not heal my fractured sense of self.

Seeds falling on barren soil.

They had no real lasting impact because of my own unguarded thoughts. Those thoughts ran like background noise, *unawares*, in spite of my early exposure to, and appreciation for, consciousness work and meditation. They were like a malware virus in my unconscious.

Brian Grasso, the author of the foreword to this book, along with his wife Carrie Campbell, founded the Mindset Performance Institute in 2014. I first heard his name in 2010, when I saw it listed among the authors of a textbook for the International Youth Conditioning Association's High School Strength & Conditioning Coach certification. Brian founded the IYCA and eventually sold it.

I saw him on Facebook a couple years later and sent him a friend request. When he announced his Mindset Performance venture and opened up enrollment for its Level 1 course, I jumped on it.

Everything I read and heard from this man resonated. I told him once I have a highly sensitive bullshit detector and not once did the needle ever move. Everything about the Institute and the coursework had me convinced I couldn't miss out. The fog of woe was lifting. I was gradually coming back to life. While still mired in my mediocrity, I was feeling hopeful, and it felt like I was turning a corner. I remember invoking Paul Newman's character in the 1982 movie, *The Verdict:*

"This is the case, there are no other cases."

I thought, "This is the course. There are no other courses." It felt like a now-or-never moment.

So often times it happens that we live our lives in chains, and we never even know we have the key."

—The Eagles, "Already Gone"

My unguarded thoughts were of stories about who I was and how I saw myself. They reflected beliefs—again, mostly unconscious; at times "semi-conscious"—about my sense of worth, what I deserved, or, more to the point, what I didn't deserve, based on some assessment of my relationship with Life, the Universe, God, Karma.

My interpretation of events, experiences, and circumstances, starting in childhood, created themes that grew in their perniciousness throughout adulthood; themes of being defective, unlovable, undeserving, *not good enough.* I was able to identify a handful of events that went a long way in creating these beliefs, this view of self.

To be clear, **and this is important,** I did not suffer the extreme trauma or abuse that often results in a wounded spirit like mine. I never blamed anyone other than myself for my struggles. The death of too many people, of close friends and family, certainly played a role. No doubt being eight years old at a time when my mother had an invalid daughter (after my sister was left paralyzed in the aftermath of her brain tumor operation) *and* an infant child to attend to can create a dynamic at odds with healthy emotional development.

I will spare you the details, but I had a couple heartbreaking disappointments resulting from some rather shitty treatment by not one but two coaches, which robbed me of the chance to play both baseball and football for my high school.

Not being from the right neighborhood seemed to be my biggest sin. This is something that came up in counseling eighteen years later. I realized then, for the first time really, just how sad I felt about it, how much it hurt, and how wronged I felt. "Not good enough" was the message I heard—not my athletic skills, but *me,* the person. I wasn't good enough.

"Everyone you meet is fighting a battle you know nothing about. Be Kind. Always."

—Unknown/Various sources

It's not anyone's place to judge another's suffering. We know neither the origins nor the nature of another person's inner struggles.

"If we could read the secret history of our enemies, we should find in each man's life sorrow and suffering enough to disarm all hostility."

—Henry Wadsworth Longfellow

###

In the nineties, I worked for yet another small personal training studio. There I met and worked with Michael O'Harro, one of the pioneers in the singles bar business. In 1983, he co-founded Champions Sports Bar in Georgetown, launching a new industry. He became known as "the Father of the Sports Bar." I trained Denyce Graves there, the famous mezzo-soprano opera singer.

The most memorable client, however, was an art teacher at Washington & Lee High School named Tucker Freeman. He asked me if I played pool. Similar to my response to Dallas about baseball, I told him I shot a good bit growing up and while in the service, but not since. He invited me to go shoot with him across the highway at a place called Cool Hands.

I fell in love with the game all over again, but this time I would become mildly obsessed with it. I wanted to learn to *really shoot pool*, not just poke and hope like the typical causal player. I knew the *game* of pool. I wanted to learn the *sport*. I wanted to learn English, position play, strategy. So, I joined a league, played competitively, and hired professional instructors.

Actually, to say pool was a mild obsession is putting it, well, mildly. On weekends, I would hit one pool hall around 7:00, play until 2:00 a.m. closing time, then drive twenty minutes to a twenty-four-hour hall and play another few hours. It became an escape. It became a therapy. It would prove to be cathartic; a crucible in which I worked out my anger, pain, frustration, and disappointment, one rack, one shot, at a time.

And it also turned out to be one of the most remarkable mindfulness meditations. The requirement of being in the moment, being so intensely present the instant the shot is taken, getting conscious to the mental commentary that can adversely affect performance—no activity turned as bright a spotlight on the impact of my thoughts as pool did. The accuracy of the shot is highly susceptible to the slightest interference from mental chatter; the feedback is immediate and obvious.

A light was slowly coming on for me. I was catching a glimpse of how all this could be applied everywhere else in life.

Somewhere around 1995, I read a book titled, *If You Meet The Buddha On the Road, Kill Him!: The Pilgrimage of Psychotherapy Patients.* Soon after, I learned that the author, Sheldon Kopp, lived and practiced in Washington, D.C. I contacted him and scheduled a session.

I don't remember much about this experience, but I do recall he was old and gray and just a tad taciturn. What I will never forget, however, is his kicking me out in the first few minutes of one of our early sessions.

My state of mind and my situation were at their worst up to that point. I said, "I need a miracle."

Not sure specifically what he said in response, but he kicked me out. He told me to get the hell out! Can you imagine that—being "fired" by your own therapist?!

"Until you make the unconscious conscious, it will direct your life and you will call it fate."

—Carl Jung

I first heard that Jung quote from Brian Grasso while enrolled in his Mindset Performance training. It speaks to why, in spite of all our conscious thoughts, words, and actions around the things we want to have and do, they often elude (many of) us. The unconscious has been busy building biases for our stories, and since these stories run counter to our conscious expression, we engage in self-defeating behavior, in self-sabotage. We look for evidence that confirms our *unconscious* beliefs. We'll even create it.

Because my beliefs of being "damaged goods," of not deserving happiness or success, were so entrenched in my unconscious, everything that didn't go right, that didn't work out for me, became a personal slight and served as further confirmation. I believe anxiety is in large part the result of unguarded thoughts, unconscious fears that create a foreboding about a world we believe is out to get us, to punish us, mock us, thwart us. Self-recrimination had become a way of life for me.

###

"WHAT ARE YOU PRETENDING NOT TO KNOW?"

"What Are You Pretending Not To Know?"

"What Are You Pretending Not To Know?"

"What are you pretending not to know?"

THIS CAN BE can be a powerful question. It's one that was on a small sign, maybe three feet in length, above the stage on the first day of the Lifespring training I did in the mid-eighties.

On day two, there it was again, only this time a litter bigger. By the final day, it was on a banner about thirty feet long.

We are masters of denial, of self-delusion. When it comes to our struggles, our lack of fulfillment, lack of success, our fruitless efforts at exercise, weight loss, and sound nutrition—we know more, often *much* more, than we let on. Why ***don't*** we do the single most effective thing to ensure good health and reduce the risk of our bodies' falling apart?? This is a perfect situation to apply that question.

For me, one of the most critical occasions to ask this question is when I am angry, at times when I've lost, or almost lost, my temper. Our own anger, if we can muster the courage to investigate it, is one of *the* most effective teachers we have. Often anger is masking pain. Anger is an expression of that pain. Most of the time, I'm angry at myself. I'm lashing out at the pain of deep disappointment.

"Every part of our personality that we do not love will become hostile to us."

—Robert Bly

"We have to face the pain we've been running from. In fact, we need to learn to rest in it and let its searing power transform us."

—Charlotte Joko Beck

One of the most powerful exercises in the Mindset Performance course, perhaps *the* most powerful, was one in which I had to list as many "self-limiting beliefs" as I could. These are beliefs that live mostly in the unconscious, but evidence of them surfaces in our self-talk often enough.

This took some unflinching self-reflection and a great deal of *not pretending* I didn't know. Since I am pretty much putting it all out there, let me share a few of them. They are in no particular order... well, except the first one...

I will never write my book.

I will never feel like I know enough professionally.

I will never feel deserving.

I will never feel whole or healed.

I will never overcome the self-defeating behaviors associated with an addictive personality.

I will never feel comfortable and confident enough to speak in front of a large group. (With small groups, I'm good)

I will never become a speaker/presenter at fitness conferences.

I will never forgive myself for not stopping to see my brother two weeks prior to his suicide or for missing his very last email.

I will never forgive myself for how I screwed up my relationship with Shelly and how that led her to getting involved with someone who may have played a role in her death.

There were more, but you get the point.

I interpreted most everything in my life through the lens of these limiting beliefs. I took more notice of the things that confirmed them.

Around 2007, a good friend and longtime client referred a friend of his to me. Peter wanted to begin training in order to fulfill his dream of climbing Mt Kilimanjaro. Our challenge was we had less than ten months to get ready and we were starting with a "sedentary, middle-aged (fifty-seven, I think he was) man carrying a few extra pounds."

We worked in his basement with a treadmill, a step-up box, and some dumbbells. On occasion, we'd load up a small backpack with twenty-five pounds or so and go to Great Falls Park on the Virginia side of the Potomac River for some hiking. Peter was consistent, determined, and he worked hard.

When the time came, we were pretty confident that he was in good enough shape to summit. And summit he did. He sent me a photo from the top of the African continent, holding a small, handwritten sign that read, "THANKS STEVE." It was one of the most gratifying experiences of my entire life—to help someone achieve a lifelong dream. It was awesome. I was so happy for him, so proud of him.

We didn't continue training after his Kilimanjaro trip. Within the next year, I got word he had been diagnosed with cancer. Less than a year after that, he was gone.

"The trouble is you think you have time."

In 2005, I met Matt Branam. He had had a "less than satisfactory" experience with one of our trainers. He contacted our corporate office and asked who our best trainer was. They gave him my name.

Matt was fifty-one at the time. He was retired. He literally started his career in the proverbial mailroom at UPS in 1973 at the age of nineteen. He worked his way up to and through management to eventually become a senior executive. When UPS went public in 1999, Matt's financial independence was assured. After UPS, he worked for a time with Elizabeth Dole, as COO at the American Red Cross.

Matt had initially intended to work with me only until the few sessions he'd rolled over from his previous trainer were used up. However, my approach was a departure from what he'd expected. He learned much more from me than he thought he would and decided to continue on.

We trained for several months consistently, and then it became more sporadic. He traveled a good bit—

Matt had a boat in the British Virgin Islands he fancied more than the gym. We ended up becoming very good friends. Matt was one of my favorite people, just a special human being. They call them "bromances," these days.

Early on, we were talking and the subject of pool came up. He told me he had a pool table at the house (it turned out he had *two* pool tables) and invited me out to shoot one night.

I pulled up to his 10,000-square-foot home in Great Falls. Holy shit! In the "great room" was a nine-foot, drop-pocket Brunswick. It came with the house. The other table he'd owned prior to moving there, a smaller one for his kids. It was clear he didn't shoot much.

He knew that, at the time, I was renting, sharing a small house with a converted attic space for a bedroom. His place had an in-law suite adjacent to this huge room.

"I don't know what you pay for rent where you are now, Steven, but I've got all this space..." He hadn't even finished making the offer but I knew where he was going.

"Hell yeah!" I said. For a few more bucks a month, I got to move into the in-law apartment, and the entire great room was mine as well, with two pool tables, ping pong and foosball tables, and a big sunken seating area with a monster-size big-screen TV.

I cherished our friendship: our substantive conversations over coffee at Greenberry's, rock concerts, ball games. Then, in 2009, for various reasons, Matt came out of retirement and took the job as president of his alma mater, the Rose-Hulman Institute of Technology in Terre Haute, Indiana. This was a five-year gig for Matt. He decided shortly thereafter to sell his house, my "home."

STEVEN HEAD

We kept in touch. I would see him when he came back to the area, where his kids still lived. In early April 2012, I got a call from him. He was in town and had a couple hours before he needed to head to the airport. We met for lunch at Kazan's, a Turkish restaurant just up from our coffee shop haunt.

He looked good; he was really enjoying his work at the school but was certain he'd be stepping down after the fifth year. We had our usual engaging conversation. We talked about how we'd resume our talks over coffee, take in some Nats games, maybe get me down to BVI and go sailing. I told him I really looked forward to all of it, and then we yelled a couple things back and forth as he walked his way to his car.

Three weeks later, Matt walked into his office on a Friday morning and collapsed—a massive heart attack. I never saw my good friend again.

"I cried when I wrote this song. Sue me if I play too long." This brother is free. I'll be what I want to be."

—Steely Dan, "Deacon Blues"

Around 1966, Chris Saverino and his parents moved into the only house on the block with a pool. His acceptance into the gang was assured. We all spent countless hours during the summer months playing Marco Polo and pissing off his dad with our cannon balls, can openers, and bananas.

In 1981, Chris and I enrolled in a SCUBA course at Northern Virginia Community College. I never completed the open water dive portion, but Chris went on to advanced certifications and ended up making a career of it. He moved to Richmond and opened a dive shop, certifying people, and hosting dive trips all over the world.

STEVEN HEAD

In 2011, the ol' neighborhood gang buried one of its own. Chris lost a long battle with cancer, and we lost a cherished friend.

In the last six months alone, I have lost three childhood friends who did not get to see their sixtieth birthday. (Make that four within the year—RIP Mark Claxton.) Ed "Eddie" Haas actually succumbed to cancer on his sixtieth birthday last June. I've known Ed since elementary school. I had lost touch with him after high school, though I knew he was still in the area. We started hanging out about six or seven years ago, after connecting via Facebook.

We shot pool together, attended rock concerts together. We met up at Nats Park to see our hometown team (after a thirty-two-year void) play. He came out to a number of my baseball games, even riding his motorcycle all the way out to Middleburg from Fairfax, just to watch his old friend play.

A couple years ago, all bundled up on a cold April day, Ed and I met up at a Nationals Opening Day game. "Let me buy you a beer."

Ed knew I enjoyed a beer now and then. What he didn't know was I'd never, ever had one at a ball game, not in eight seasons of attending Nats games. (Typically, I've driven to the game; also, I refuse to spend eight bucks for a beer!) I told him that and then gladly accepted his offer. If I ever drink another, I will raise my bottle in a toast, to Ed.

The names I share won't mean much to most of you, but I wanted to acknowledge them, to honor them. They are a part of my story, my life. A big part. They are central to one of the most important messages of this book.

In her book, *Writing As A Way Of Healing: How Telling Our Stories Transforms Our Lives,* Louise DeSalvo notes, "People who write about their loved ones' deaths are paradoxically engaged in a search for a meaning of their loved ones' lives. They want to make a record; they want to describe their loss and their grief. But they want to discover, too, an overarching meaning for this death so it will not have been for naught. This seems especially necessary if the death was a violent one, if it was a suicide or an accident or if it was the death of a child. For these deaths greatly threaten our sense of order. They shake the foundations in our belief in a meaningful, beneficent universe; they make us question whether any actions we may take have any meaning."

You can imagine how I might have interpreted or internalized the death of so many people close to me.

I was cursed.

"If we see the suffering and wounds of our addictive life as a lesson that can be passed along to others, we can transform the wound into a gift. Having lived through a life threatening crisis, we become healers."

—Linda Leonard

So much of the deprivation and isolation I've endured over the past twenty-five years has been a self-administered punishment for all my mistakes, real and imagined; cruel and unusual punishment for my perceived shortcomings.

Though I bought into these self-defeating stories, *some part of me* always knew they were bullshit. That part, however suppressed, is what I think of as my Higher Self, or the superconscious, as it is known in some spiritual circles. This is what sustained me.

As much as I lived and acted as though I believed these stories, at a deeper level I truly did not. I had an overriding faith, a belief, even a confidence, ironically enough, that there was a purpose to all the struggle, loss, and grief. I just "knew" it would eventually give birth to a bigger, broader calling in service to others. I didn't know how or when, but I knew that "this, too, shall pass."

###

MEDITATION AT WORK

"No matter what area of your life seems to you to be blocked or thwarted, stop and reconsider: you will recognize the outer 'enemy' as but a reflection of what you have not, before now, been willing or able to recognize as coming from within."

—Ralph Blum

EARLY ON IN MY tenure (about 2005-06) at our big box gym where I'm still employed (at the time of this writing, anyway), I found myself extremely unhappy. I was frustrated, unfulfilled—you name it.

Not happy with management. Not feeling particularly appreciated. And yes, in moments of honest self-reflection, very disappointed with my station in life and what I saw as a lack of professional accomplishment. I had hit a bottom. Maybe not *the* bottom, necessarily, but I was about as unhappy and dissatisfied as I'd ever been.

"It may be that when we no longer know what to do we have come to our real work and that when we no longer know which way to go we have begun our real journey."

—Wendell Berry

"True love and prayer are learned in the hour when love becomes impossible and the heart has turned to stone."

—Thomas Merton

I wasn't happy with any aspect of my work there during this time. I don't think I'd ever been that unhappy with a work situation.

I complained a lot and felt pretty ashamed of that fact. I was even more ashamed of times when I was passive-aggressive. *Ugh.* Ugly. Though not to this degree, I'd been here before: unhappy with a job, blaming external factors for my unhappiness, and leaving to find something better.

Not this time. I realized it was my mindset, my attitudes that were making me miserable, and if I left under these circumstances, the pattern would undoubtedly repeat itself. This time, I was going to stay and find a way to love my job again, right where I was.

For a few years there, I know I wasn't much fun to be around. I was pretty miserable, and I'm sure many around me would agree! I'm certain I alienated a number of people. No doubt I owe a number of clients an apology for not giving, not being enough. Without question, I still have my lapses, occasionally falling back into old patterns.

STEVEN HEAD

"But I think it's about forgiveness, forgiveness..."
—Don Henley, "The Heart of the Matter"

In her book, *A Heart as Wide as the World: Stories on the Path of Lovingkindness,* Sharon Salzberg writes, "We cannot undo what we have done, and we cannot escape the results of our actions. But rather than hate ourselves or dwell in helpless shame, we can dramatically change the field in which our karmic seeds ripen by developing *mindfulness and lovingkindess.* (Emphasis mine.) This is the basis of a spiritual life."

Bingo.

"Heaven is right where you are standing and that is the place to practice."

—Morehei Ueshiba

"There are two ways to live your life. One as if nothing is a miracle. The other is as though everything is a miracle."

—Albert Einstein

Drawing on all that I read and learned through the years, I made a conscious decision to approach my work as a meditation. I was going to make it my spiritual practice. I would observe and guard my thoughts more. Bitch and complain less. Be less judgmental, *a lot less.* I was going to notice more, appreciate more, and pay closer attention—to everything. I was going to look people in the eye more regularly as I passed. I would smile and greet them. I was going to try to see the miracles.

Some twenty years ago, I read Dale Carnegie's classic, *How to Win Friends & Influence People*. The *one thing* I remember from it to this day is how Carnegie suggests the sweetest sound to a person's ears is the sound of their own name. I was going to meet more people, learn their names, and greet them by name. Unlike my previous two workplaces, which were small, personal training studios, this club is huge, with close to 4,000 members. I realized I had the opportunity to meet dozens of people every single day. I came to think of it as the *"Cheers* effect" (think theme song for the TV series).

One pleasant discovery I made: a number of people who, in my mind, I was sure were "jerks," when I made it a point to actually introduce myself to them, turned out to be perfectly nice people. Go figure. One of the common defense mechanisms for someone who has struggled with self-worth/esteem issues is a sort of "preemptive rejection" strategy. This is something that happens almost completely unconsciously, below the radar.

"For well you know that it's a fool, who plays it cool, by making his world a little colder."

—Lennon/McCartney

Eye contact. A smile. A "Hello." When I began to make a concerted effort to greet more people, I discovered (rediscovered?) a few things.

One, I couldn't be all in my head in my typical self-absorbed state. It required a "generosity of spirit," a willingness to extend myself. I also noticed that many people—I mean a remarkable number—did not want to make eye contact, couldn't muster a smile, and apparently had no interest in saying hello. Some would even make obvious efforts to avoid it. It was tempting to take it personally at times but I quickly realized it really had nothing to do with me.

Fortunately, there were also plenty of members who absolutely lit up when I smiled and said hello to them, especially the older ones. Many folks just wanted to be acknowledged.

"Life is not lost by dying. Life is lost in the minute by minute, day by dragging day, in all the thousand small uncaring ways."

—Stephen Vincent Benet

My work—that is my experience of it—slowly began to transform.

I decided to let go of any and all "blame," including any for myself. I made a much wiser decision: I took accountability, instead. I dropped all the bullshit stories I had told myself about why I was miserable at work. I took full responsibility for my situation. I could just as easily have become a personal trainer statistic, succumbing to burnout and leaving the industry altogether. But that "Higher Self" and its sense of a higher calling wouldn't hear of it.

I got some help and inspiration from a couple industry leaders, which helped spark a renewed passion for my work. Michael Boyle of Mike Boyle Strength & Conditioning and Mark Verstegen, founder of EXOS, formerly known as Athletes Performance Institute.

In my search to learn how to better train for performance on the baseball field, I found these two guys. Their work opened my eyes to how complacent I'd become and to the Truth (with a capital T) of famous coach John Wooden's statement, "It's what you learn *after* you know it all that really matters."

"What is necessary to create change is to change one's awareness of self."

—Abraham Maslow

It's been twelve years now since my "mid-career crisis." That alone is roughly two times as long as the average personal trainer's entire *career*. In that time, I've worked with hundreds of folks, mostly in the fifty- to seventy-year-old range.

Many came to me with chronic pain issues, lingering injuries, and a host of stories about what they couldn't do anymore. They came with misconceptions and misinformation about exercise. But more importantly, they came; they showed up. They came with a degree of trust and maybe with a prodding from their own "higher self," sensing that with some guidance they could tap the potential waiting inside. I hope to offer some of that guidance in Part 2, the "manual" part of this book.

I'm no miracle worker, as I've had to remind a client or two on occasion! But what I do see as a miracle, be it of divine origin or otherwise, is our body. And it has become quite clear to me that *movement* was inherent in the grand design. The fact that exercise is as close to

[126]

a panacea as there is, as close to a fountain of youth as it gets, speaks to the fundamental role that consistent, challenging movement plays in our health.

THIS is where that higher calling lies for me. This book, however small its impact may be, is a start. My generation has been sold a bill of goods, duped by pharmaceutical companies and a complicit medical industry into accepting pain and debility as normal, as a natural consequence of aging. Further confounding the issue is my industry itself, with too much of it relying on the "PT Barnum School of Marketing." Even many legitimate professionals, in an effort to stand out in a noisy, crowded marketplace, muddy the waters by endlessly debating minutiae and sending out conflicting messages to a public that can't make heads or tails of it all.

Depending on which part of the elephant (the fitness industry) *this* blind man is describing, it appears far too many are trying to outdo each other and make a name for themselves among their peers and colleagues, all while Rome burns. Way too much of fitness marketing is sexualized, further suggesting it is the exclusive domain of the young.

It's a bit of a paradox that exercise science is both at once complex and yet fundamentally rather simple. There is no shortage of rabbit holes to crawl down, for those inclined; no end to the minutiae one can get mired in. I get it: for our profession to be taken seriously, we have to be vigilant in our efforts to be guided by science, by evidence. The envelope must be pushed to advance sports performance, as well as to refine and update what works on the fitness floor.

That said, if we are to lower the "barriers of entry" for those sitting on the sidelines, then the message has to be simplified. I am primarily concerned with average folks, boomers specifically, whose health may already be failing due to years of sedentary living, who are on a laundry list of medications, whose joints are failing, and who have been convinced (with some complicitness for sure) that fitness is too complicated, too demanding, or too extreme for folks their age. There are roughly forty-nine million of us!

To hell with that.

I want to [help] make America strong and healthy again. I want to be part of a campaign that gets this message out there on a bigger, wider scale.

"Unite the Clans!"

—William Wallace in *Braveheart*

Depression. Diabetes. "Bad" backs. "Bad" knees. Chronic pain. Treating the side effects of a drug with more drugs. Falling prey to quick-fix promises. We are better than this!

With health care such as it is, including high insurance premiums, drug costs, etc., it's time we as a nation, and baby boomers especially, take a good hard look at exercise (formal and informal activity) as a means to staying out the doctor's office, the operating room, and the line at the pharmacy. I want to inspire people, to convince them exercise can actually be *enjoyable* and the benefits afforded are within their reach and well worth the effort, accessible to anyone.

"It is a shame for a man to grow old without seeing the beauty and strength of which his body is capable."

—Plato

###

OUR "WHY"

"The reason I exercise is for the quality of life I enjoy."
—Dr. Kenneth Cooper

IF YOU'VE HUNG IN this far, my sincere thanks for letting me share my story with you.

One of the most often recommended books in my circle is actually about business and leadership: Simon Sinek's *Start with Why*. I have articulated or alluded to a few of my whys. Exercise has helped me manage and overcome severe depression. It has enabled me to get out and enjoy the beauty of the wilderness and the mountains, on foot and not merely on my ass from the seat of a car. So, I've stuck with it, hoping to serve as a role model, encouraging others.

I have taken on clients in their late fifties, sixties, even seventies, with either "bad knees" or a "bad" back or both, with a history of fits and starts in the gym. I've seen many of them work the process to emerge strong, *empowered,* and free of pain. They've gone on to achieve strength levels they never imagined, along with other newfound or regained abilities.

My whys even include a sense of civic duty. I do not want to be part of the crushing burden that frail, ailing boomers are putting on, and will continue to put on, our health care system and our economy. The more I can avoid relying on expensive and often inefficient health care, the better. Physical independence, mobility, and the ability to carry out activities of daily living—that's what's at stake.

When I was in massage school (1996), one of our assignments was to visit a nursing home, offer massage to residents, and then write up our experience. Most folks welcomed the company; the massage was little more than a caring touch, a holding, or a stroking of their hand. I wrote in my summary I couldn't shake the thought of how many of these folks hadn't had regular exercise in their life, and if they'd had, might they have avoided or at least forestalled their current "predicament?"

"The preservation of health is a duty. Few seem conscious that there is such a thing as physical morality."

—Herbert Spencer

It is estimated that 80% of Americans believe in God, yet how many of us "glorify God" in our bodies? (1 Corinthians 6:20)

My commitment to exercise is a form of reverence, of prayer, of gratitude. It allowed me to rediscover my childhood love of baseball and to play it now for two decades. Every time I take the field, I literally pinch myself on the thigh and send a thought up to my dad.

Knock wood, I am on zero medications. Other than the single three-month prescription of Prozac and an antibiotic on a handful of occasions, I've been med-free my entire adult life. I've had clients who, over time, were able to wean themselves off most of and, in a few cases, their entire laundry list.

"All parts of the body ... if used in moderation and exercised in labors in which each is accustomed become thereby healthy, well developed and age slowly, but if unused and left idle they become liable to disease and age quickly."

—Hippocrates

What might be your "WHY?"

It's worth asking yourself, if it applies, "Why *don't* I exercise?" If one is honest with oneself, and investigates the answers, it can be powerful. However, even more powerful would be to discover WHYs that inspire you to move, to commit to exercise. Can you think of a higher purpose of your own that being strong, fit, and capable could serve? Volunteer work? Maybe active, adventurous vacations with your spouse? Rediscovering a childhood joy? Playing with your grandkids? A much-needed, much-deserved practice of self-love?

In the following pages, I want to offer some insight and information in the hopes of keeping your hows from getting in the way of your whys!

###

STEVEN HEAD

PART 2
A Memoir-esque Manual

###

STEVEN HEAD

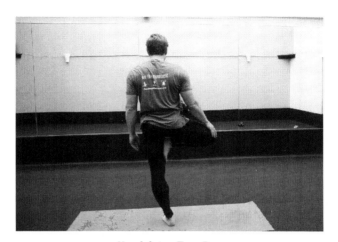

Head doing Tree Pose

THE PSYCHOLOGICAL MINE FIELD

INFORMATION. There is certainly no shortage of it. If information were all we needed, we'd all be fit. Intellect? Most of us are smart enough to recognize we should exercise, *should* move more, in order to be healthier. You would've had to be living under a rock for a couple decades to not be aware of the myriad health benefits associated with regular exercise. When you aren't "pretending not to know," *you likely know what they are*!

Folks who just love exercise, those committed to an active lifestyle, are in the vast *minority*. When one works in the industry and when the vast *majority* of one's Facebook friends are fellow industry professionals, it's easy to forget that at times.

Why is this true? Why do so few of us take care of ourselves with the single most effective means we have at our disposal? Intellectually, it's a no-brainer. But yet there is so much that conspires to keep us sedentary. Our very culture militates against us moving. There's so much that has us convinced (and too many of us were convinced too easily) we can't be one of those fit folks who actually enjoys exercise. As I alluded to early on, the biggest obstacles are of our own making, the result of what goes on in our head, and too much of that goes on unchecked.

I know a great deal about getting in my own way, though it's been a decades-long process of becoming conscious to it. The damage, the cost: incalculable. Fitness is about the only area of my life spared from self-defeating behavior. This portion of the book is to help you get out of your own way.

Gray Cook, a physical therapist, strength coach, and one of the most brilliant minds in the industry, authored what has become a mantra, a guiding principle: "First, move well, and then, move often." I suggest there's a prerequisite of sorts for many of us: "First, learn how and why you are in your own way, and then move out of the way!" It's a notion not dissimilar to the wisdom contained in Abraham Lincoln's quote, "If I had six hours to cut down a tree, I'd spend the first four hours sharpening the axe."

"Fitness must begin in the mind, and mindfulness in the body."

—Steven Head (with inspiration from B.K.S. Iyengar)

What if I told you that you could hire a coach who would work with you for free as frequently as you wanted/needed, would do so without judgment, would support you with unconditional love, and help you see things you are too close to see for yourself; one who could prevent you from getting in your own way, would never lose patience with you, and would help you develop the tools and skills to give you the best chance at success for incorporating "movement medicine" into your life? Would you be interested? Gosh, I would sure hope so!

"All men should strive to learn before they die, what they are running from, and to, and why."

—James Thurber

That coach is *you.* But the only way to be that coach for yourself is to slow down, quit running, and be still.

Ironic, huh? This is the sharpening of the axe. For those who don't currently exercise, *this might be the best place to start.* The insight, skills, and wisdom garnered here will fell the tree.

I'm going to try to distill in just a few pages what I've come to know through years of personal experience, dozens of books read, a number of courses taken, as well as observing hundreds and hundreds of clients through the lens of mindfulness. Not easy. I hope to present the practice of mindfulness and meditation in a way so as to dispel some misconceptions, create a modicum of understanding, and spark an interest in further exploration and discovery.

While not another fitness book, this is not intended to be an exhaustive treatise on mindfulness and meditation, either. Again, it's my hope that you, the reader, are ready when this book shows up. I'm planting a seed. I hope you will water it.

[143]

I began teaching yoga in 1997. I teach it as a meditative art, as a mindfulness practice that uses the poses as tools for improving body awareness, mental concentration, and emotional equanimity. Over the years, I've had numerous conversations about people's perceptions of it and experiences with it.

Some of the more common disparaging remarks I heard were along the lines of, "Oh I can't do yoga, too boring."

"Too slow."

"I just can't be that still."

"Tried it *once,* drove me crazy."

"Yoga's not for me, I'm too stiff, not flexible." (That last one kills me.)

This offers a glimpse into our predicament. For so many of us, slowing down, sitting still, paying attention to our breath, and observing our thoughts without distractions seems unbearable. To make matters worse we are so ego-defended that we can't (aren't willing to) recognize what the benefit would be. And it's in large part because of this that our efforts to begin and establish a fit lifestyle are often doomed from the start.

Stay with me.

Pop quiz:

- ✓ Have you ever walked into a room and forgotten why you went in?
- ✓ Have you ever driven past your exit?
- ✓ Have you ever been introduced to someone and within moments can't "remember" their name?
- ✓ Ever noticed a construction site along a *regularly traveled* route where a building has been razed, but for the life of you, you can't remember what was there?

✓ Have you ever been unable to find your keys when you *just* had them two minutes ago?

✓ How is it you can find something somewhere that, when you looked in the exact same place just a minute earlier, you did not see?

These are just a few relatively innocuous examples of lapses in awareness or attention, situations in which we were lost in thought. Being lost in thought is the antithesis of mindfulness. *And herein lies the rub*: we are lost in thought so much of our lives. Many of our waking hours are spent ruminating about the past or fretting about the future or otherwise preoccupied with someone or something, all of which compromises our experience of the present.

Almost cliché, right? The very fact that it sounds cliché to many is itself symptomatic of our tendency to dismiss some of the most fundamental and powerful truths because they just seem too simple, not sexy enough. To make matters worse, media overexposure can turn a powerful practice into a platitude. Magazine articles, news stories, etc. about mindfulness seem to be everywhere these days. When something reaches such pop-culture popularity, it becomes easy to dismiss without ever really understanding it.

Our thoughts are, for the most part, habitual, repetitive, and constant. Many of them are driven and distorted by our emotions, fears, insecurities, and desires, and as long as we remain unaware of them, as long as we never investigate them, never question, never challenge them, our thoughts *will* have *us*, and our emotions *will have us,* and *not* the other way around.

We have opinions about everything and, too often, take our opinions to be fact. We believe everything we think and *rarely, if ever,* question. We make assumptions and believe them. We make predictions as forgone conclusions about how things will go or be. We label, we categorize and judge *constantly.*

In our labeling, categorizing, and judging, we establish our "certainty" about things. We get to think, "I know." We relieve the angst of not knowing because uncertainty and not knowing are just too damn uncomfortable; intolerable for many of us.

That's what we humans do, *all of us*, to varying degrees.

Unfortunately, in our haste to eliminate uncertainty, in our need to (think we) know, we cut off further inquiry, never revisit or question, and we miss out on the possibility of more precise, more accurate knowledge. We fall victim to hasty conclusions. This is so much a thing, it's referred to by psychologists as "premature cognitive commitment."

> *"We would rather be ruined than changed.*
> *We would rather die in our dread*
> *than to climb the cross of the moment*
> *and let our illusions die."*
> —W.H. Auden, *The Age of Anxiety*

"Until you are willing to be confused about what you already know, what you know will never grow bigger, better or more useful."

—Milton Erikson

Numerous times each day, I catch myself being mindless. I'm reminded to not be hard on myself. Having space to "fail" is critical. Compassion, something we could all use more of, must begin at home. I realize every waking second, I am vulnerable to this propensity for mindlessness and to getting lost in thought. I found this story about Socrates in Dr. Kabot-Zinn's *Full Catastrophe Living* (that seminal book I mentioned earlier).

"Socrates was famous in Athens for saying, 'Know thyself.' It is said that one of his students asked him: 'Socrates you go around saying, "Know thyself," but do you know yourself?' Socrates replied, 'No, but I understand something about this not knowing.'"

"All man's miseries derive from not being able to sit in a quiet room alone."

—Blaise Pascal

Nothing esoteric about it. Nothing religious about it. Nothing mystical about it. Nothing particularly complicated about it. While it *is* simple as a concept, actually living it is a bit more challenging. Establishing a practice will push us right up against everything that has had us on the run. Some of what we discover about ourselves, what we get conscious to, is not particularly flattering; some of it may be downright unsettling. The good news is, quite often, if we can manage to step out of the rush and compulsion of everyday doing, we can experience something quite profound: the joy of being okay with *just being*.

"Be still, and know that I am God."

—Psalm 46:10

"We have to try to cure our faults by attention and not by will."

—Simone Weil

We sit and turn our awareness to our breath, which serves as our anchor to the present moment. The breath becomes slower, fuller, and we elicit the relaxation response (please Google it, if you haven't yet). As your mind wanders, and it most certainly will, you'll eventually realize you've lost awareness of your breath and wandered away from the present moment. This is also critical: it doesn't matter how often that happens, because each and every time you bring your awareness back to your breath, you have trained yourself in the skill of being present and of *being in your body.*

Perhaps the most common misconception I hear about meditation is the erroneous belief that the goal is to turn off one's thoughts, to "clear the mind." Good luck with that! Impossible. No, the "goal" is to become conscious to our thought life, to the incessant nature of our thoughts, and to the content, the emotional energy surrounding those thoughts. As we return again and again to the breath, what may happen is, with practice the calm, quiet space between thoughts may lengthen a bit and we may spend a little less time lost in those thoughts.

If you have any doubts about this, any doubt about how undisciplined your ordinary consciousness is, try this: sit for just five minutes, doing nothing, but trying to stay conscious of your breath. As you notice it slowing down, try to count ten conscious, *unhurried* breaths.

Try it now.

There's a high probability that, somewhere before the third or fourth breath, your mind already wandered off and you lost count.

We undertake this practice to create a much keener awareness of the constant, habituated chatter going on in our own mind. *Unless we slow down, stop, and sit to observe our thoughts, we'll never learn the extent to which we are controlled and tyrannized by them.* That awareness is actually made possible by becoming an objective, *non-judgmental* observer to the nature of all that damn thinking. Assuming the stance of an impartial witness to it over time enables us to create some distance, some detachment from them. We slowly become *less* reactive to them, *less* identified with them, *less* controlled by them. And, in this case, less is so much more.

This is HUGE.

In time, you learn you can have thoughts and not react to them. You learn, between a stimulus (an event, a thought) and the otherwise knee-jerk response, you now have the ability, the freedom, to choose either a non-reaction or a more skillful, wiser, calmer response. This freedom is fundamental to the teachings of Buddhism on wisdom and the minimization of needless suffering.

It is no accident, in his book, Kabot-Zinn lists Non-Judging as the first attitude under "The Attitudinal Foundation of Mindfulness Practice." I think it's worth mentioning again that Kabot-Zinn's book is 444 pages and covers, in detail, his program at the University of Massachusetts Medical Center, a program that has operated for forty years using mindfulness-based meditation and yoga (real yoga, not the bastardized versions rampant in health clubs across the country) as its only interventions to help patients cope with chronic stress, anxiety, pain, and illness.

How does this relate to exercise? Glad you asked. If we choose to do so, we can step back, become aware of, and challenge our judgments.

Do you have judgments about how hard exercise is? Do you have negative judgments about your abilities or lack thereof? What about the time commitment, about how boring it seems, about how complicated it appears? Maybe we'll come to realize just how much we've been manipulated, duped by our judging mind. Stories! So much of what we think, of what we tell ourselves, of what we act on as though it were actually true, is just fucking stories! We can have these thoughts, recognize them as nothing more, and realize they may not even be the truth and we have the freedom *to not act on them.*

[155]

There are a couple types of judging thoughts that are particularly insidious and subversive. So much so, in fact, that, thousands of years ago, in the Buddhist tradition, they were recognized as obstacles to spiritual enlightenment. These two, along with three others, are known as the Five Kleshas (*klesha* translates to poison), i.e., negative mental states or afflictions that create suffering. Getting conscious to these and their sway over us will go a very long way to improving our chances of exercise success. They are known as Attachment (or Desire) and Aversion.

When I suggested our thoughts and emotions *have us,* rather than the other way around, I had these in mind. They are so common and "subtle," they usually go unnoticed. Thoughts and statements that start out, "I wish...," "I hate...," "He always...," and "She never...," offer clues into how much we are at the mercy of our attachments and aversions. Compulsive, chronic complaining—the room's too warm, too cold. Damn

[156]

traffic. Long, slow checkout line. You get the idea. "First-world problems."

Obviously, there is nothing wrong or abnormal about having likes and dislikes. That's not the point. Again, it's the lack of awareness around them that is at issue. There's a saying that goes, "Pain is inevitable, suffering is optional." This speaks to how attached we are to having everything go our way, and how averse we are to inconveniences, discomfort, and disappointments. Life is uncomfortable and, at times, painful. Suffering is what we heap on top of that pain, on top of the discomfort and disappointment, *according to our degree* of attachment and aversion.

"Men are disturbed, not by things, but by the principles and notions which they form concerning things."

—Epictetus

I've seen the above quote translated, "Men aren't so much disturbed by things as they are by their opinion about things." Our opinions are often expressions of our attachments and aversions. The Buddha spoke of the inevitable experience of pain, discomfort, and inconvenience as the "First dart." The suffering comes when we, ourselves, throw the "Second dart."

###

We exhibit tendencies towards attachment and aversion, almost addict-like, to our comforts, our conveniences, to things going our way, to our likes and dislikes. This "addiction-esque" behavior also shows up in our constant need for stimulation, distraction, and activity. Attachment and aversion are very much two sides of the same coin.

According to a 2015 Surgeon General's report, an estimated twenty-one million Americans suffer with substance addiction. If we throw in a half-dozen or so socially sanctioned addictions (e.g., gambling, sex/porn, shopping, Internet, tobacco, smart phones), we've got a substantial portion of the population exhibiting addictive behavior.

Though we may not be addicts in the classic or medical sense, many of us are, in fact, addicted. The addict is running *from* pain (Aversion), typically emotional, and running *to* (Attachment) an escape, a high, or a sense pleasure, for temporary relief from that pain. The addiction model offers some insight into, and understanding of, our own restlessness, our inability to ground ourselves and just be. It gives us a glimpse into why we struggle to stay centered and tolerate the discomfort (often mischaracterized as pain) inherent in exercise. It can offer a glimpse into why we find it difficult to tolerate the *perceived* tedium of physical activity or formal exercise.

Exercise, by definition, requires some exertion. If we cannot see our attachment and aversion surrounding this fact—that exercise involves some discomfort—then our judging, unchecked thoughts can make it very difficult to accept and overcome.

"When running up a hill, it is all right to give up as many times as you wish—as long as you keep your feet moving."

—Shoma Morita, M.D.

###

In the twenty-plus years I've been teaching yoga, I've been asked numerous times why I don't play music in class. The reason is it would be just another concession

[160]

to people's attachment to or dependence on external stimuli. It would represent yet another distraction, as subtle as it might be.

Historically, yoga was a comprehensive system for spiritual growth. There were eight limbs that comprised what is known as Ashtanga Yoga. The poses, which we may have some familiarity with, are but one of the eight. Another one of the limbs is pratyahara, which is the withdrawing of the senses, a pulling back from external stimuli that bombard us constantly nowadays. Think about how much of the day you are exposed to outside noise—from the TV, radio, traffic, the Internet. Walking the grocery store aisles, we get pitched via the PA system. Hell, these days you can't even pump your gas in peace: there are speakers in the ceilings or monitors in the pumps broadcasting the news or an enticement to come inside and buy a cup of coffee and a doughnut.

I was recently reminded just how pervasive this auditory assault is. At one of my favorite venues,

Nationals (Baseball) Park, not a single otherwise silent moment is left unmolested by music, announcements, games on the Jumbotron, or some other form of entertainment between innings. Even in the few seconds between pitches, they manage to blast out a song snippet. God forbid we should be left to fend for ourselves, *from* ourselves.

Silence and solitude have become rare experiences. Both are hard to come by, and they're just too scary for many of us, yet they are so very salutary. When you get in your car, do you immediately turn on the radio? This can be a mindfulness moment. I *love* music, and I like to listen to the news (though I am growing weary of it lately). I purposely, deliberately, make the decision during some point in my trip to turn off the radio and enjoy the silence.

You can create your own mindfulness reminders beyond "taking the one seat" (formal, seated meditation), like during your morning shower or some other activity you do every day. No doubt your mind in the shower is chattering away about this, that, or the other thing. Make it a point to just quiet it down with your breath and turn your awareness to the water hitting your skin, to the sound the water makes. Choose one or two activities to serve as a reminder to get present and just breathe. Over time, the mind will begin to "automatically" remind you when you begin that activity.

Between attachment and aversion lives this thing called "acceptance." Acceptance is not resignation, nor is it surrender. It is "merely" a wise choice to not force or fight what already is.

Because, fortunately...

"Everything in life that we really accept undergoes a change."

—Katherine Mansfield

Acceptance is a necessary prerequisite to desired change. Every January, I see new members join the gym. Many seem to fight and try to force through their lack of acceptance of their current state. These are typically the ones who disappear by mid-February.

Five minutes. Let's face it, the excuse/story that we don't have time for something, be it meditation or exercise, is just about the biggest lie we perpetrate on ourselves. If you are willing to sit for little more than the length of a typical commercial break, you may be blown away by what you discover. Spend five minutes bringing awareness back to the breath as often as needed and observe the thoughts as they come and go.

Boredom? Physical pain or discomfort? Restlessness? Anxiousness? Calm? Serenity? Judging? Any or all of it? Good. You did it right.

There really is no other goal than to just notice what you notice, *without judgment*. In time, the mindfulness cultivated in those five minutes can carry over into the rest of the day, and life itself becomes a more meditative experience. We become more present, and the ordinary can become more extraordinary. Your breath is always with you, always available to anchor your awareness to, to calm your body and mind.

"The real voyage of discovery consists not in seeking new landscapes, but in having new eyes."

—Marcel Proust

With advancing age, life is too often reduced to a two-dimensional imposter of the real thing, with our lifelong habits of thought and action on a continuous loop. Ever notice how "old folks" (many; not all, of course) repeat the same stories, tell the same jokes, and have canned, stock responses to similar situations? Ever notice how little old folks notice? The depth of our awareness and the richness of our experience as we advance in age can become like a flat stone skipping across the surface of a small pond clear to the other side, never penetrating the surface.

It doesn't have to be that way. With what science is learning about the positive effects exercise has on the brain and the brain's neuroplasticity, the combination of mindfulness and movement can go a long way to keeping our minds sharp as we age.

In spite of all the media coverage and hype surrounding the practice of mindfulness and meditation, many have never read a book or an article on the subject, let alone attempted to practice it. If I have convinced or inspired you to give mindfulness practice and meditation a try, a word of caution. Just like the new gym member in January, who is brimming with enthusiasm for their New Year's commitment to exercise, we need to temper our zeal, should we decide to take up the practice.

If we go in thinking it's going to be some kind of miracle cure, we are sure to be disappointed. On the flip side, if we are cynical or overly skeptical, there's a good chance we'll convince ourselves meditation is of no value. Patience and practice, however, will most assuredly yield benefits. But keep in mind, there's benefit to be had the *very minute* we slow down, become conscious of our breath, step back from our thoughts, and get present.

I've had a number of folks over the years come up to me after their *first* yoga class to tell me how much better they felt—calmer, more centered, more grounded. When I have someone in my class who is new to yoga, I explain that I teach it as a meditative art, a mindfulness practice. I mention that, for some, it's seen as a spiritual practice. I follow that up by saying the most "spiritual" we get in my class is to practice with the hope of growing in self-awareness, which often leads to greater self-acceptance.

[167]

I know my practice has led me to be more patient, *far more* than I'd be otherwise. As I've grown in self-awareness, grown more conscious to my own faults, shortcomings, and "inconsistencies," I have in turn grown in self-acceptance. My patience with others is a result of that self-compassion. Quite often, I recognize myself in their behavior. Because of all this, there's far less projection on my part, far less ego-defending.

I've been giving the following notion a lot of thought lately, and it's been truly powerful. I rediscovered it thumbing through the seminal book I mentioned early on, *The Handbook to Higher Consciousness*. These days, so many folks seem on edge, easily offended, short-tempered, etc. Ken Keyes, Jr. wrote, "You add suffering to the world just as much when you take offense as when you give offense."

Think about that for a few minutes. Better yet, each time you are tempted to take offense at the slightest slight.

###

"As to methods, there may be a million and then some, but principles are few. The man who grasps principles can successfully select his own methods."

—Ralph Waldo Emerson

"Everything should be made as simple as possible. But not simpler."

—Albert Einstein

I mentioned James Joyce's "Mr. Duffy," who lived a short distance from his body. If we have spent a lifetime living in our heads with all our unguarded thoughts, we quite possibly have lost touch with our bodies. Mindfulness, which I've mentioned must begin in the body, will enable us to grow in our acceptance of that body, become more attuned to it, and become a better authority on its needs, particularly with regard to exercise. We will be less at the mercy of all the marketing manipulation and the countless, conflicting and confusing opinions. Armed with an understanding of basic principles, we can guide our training with our own intuition, our own instincts, as opposed to doing some routine over and over because all we have are a limited number of memorized methods.

Now that we know a bit about how to get out of our own way, we are ready to arm ourselves with some of those principles. We'll discuss some concepts, and I'll share some additional philosophy and opinions I've formulated over the years. I will share what I have come to believe are some of the most critical strategies for success. I also want to alert you to some of the common mindset missteps folks make when they step into the gym. Let's start there…

###

MINDSET MISSTEP # 1

NOT THINKING OUTSIDE THE BOX...

...THE BIG-BOX GYM, that is.

If exercise isn't enjoyable for us, or at least rewarding and gratifying, if it doesn't serve a higher purpose, if it's viewed only as a necessary chore, something only done in the gym on "fancy" equipment, it may not take root.

So, formal exercise should be seen as part of an overall approach that blends physical activity (e.g.,

taking stairs instead of the elevator for less than a three-
or four-floor trip; carrying groceries to the car versus
pulling the car around) with a recreational pursuit and
alternate venues for formal exercise.

For example, you could easily have a home gym that
requires minimal space and equipment. Also, office
building stairwells: climbing stairs is such great way to
get cardiovascular conditioning, develop leg and hip
strength (especially two steps at a time) and burn lots
of calories. You get all that without the impact of
running. Another idea is to visit a nearby playground
with a couple resistance bands and get a great workout.
Or an agility ladder, something you might think only
athletes employ, can be as much fun as playing
hopscotch was when you were a kid.

Learn to play again.

###

MINDSET MISSTEP # 2

TOO MUCH, TOO SOON

FAILING TO SEE EXERCISE in this broader context can lead to one of the most common self-sabotaging "strategies" there is: the "too much, too soon" and its close cousin, the "all or none." We want to be committed for the duration, for the rest of our lives. With the big picture in mind and a commitment to the long haul, we don't need to be perfect, and we don't have to be in a hurry.

[173]

One of the easiest ways to derail efforts to establish exercise as a new, permanent lifestyle change is to try to overcome decades of an old lifestyle in the first couple of weeks. If we push too hard, do too much too soon, or are sore for three days after every workout, either by our own doing or at the hands of an inexperienced, misguided trainer, we are very likely to throw in the towel, assuming we don't get injured first. To be sure, some mild muscle soreness after a workout is to be expected now and then, particularly with a new exercise or an increase in intensity with a familiar one. But it should not be debilitating, and it shouldn't last more than a day or two.

Quite often, in the first week, a new client will ask, "Is that it? That's *all*?"

I answer, "Yes." And then, I explain why. Regardless of what specific goals we have, consistency over the long haul is the only way to achieve them. That requires patience, which, in my humble opinion, is one of the highest forms of wisdom. It requires gradual increases in volume and effort in order to avoid injury, overreaching, and getting turned off to the whole idea. Our tolerance for discomfort must be allowed to slowly build up over time.

I tell new clients that goals are great, but we need to be less fixated on specific outcomes and more oriented to the process. I'll say, "Each workout must become its own reward." Results come and goals are achieved with a commitment to the process.

Nothing beats consistency. Nothing. If we expect unreasonable results or results unreasonably quickly, we will be frustrated and disappointed.

###

STEVEN HEAD

S&M: STRONG & MOBILE

THESE TWO CAPACITIES should probably be the focus of anyone who takes up exercise, be it for health, fat loss (yes, fat loss), appearance, or performance. Even those who have an endurance activity goal in mind (e.g., an obstacle course run, long bike ride, a 5K or 10K run) would benefit greatly from improvements to both. (They would, of course, do more cardio/aerobic endurance training, in addition.) Strength and mobility will make us all more durable for anything, from activities of daily living (ADLs) to more ambitious physical pursuits.

[176]

To be strong: who wouldn't want that? Think about it. So, why is it so many of us are what I've come to refer to as "strength-o-phobes?" Many women, old *and* young fear lifting weights will make them bulky and less feminine. This, pardon me for saying so, is a bit silly.

Men and women both, especially those north of fifty, are often overly concerned, needlessly so, with getting hurt. A large number of the orthopedic problems that beset us baby boomers can be linked to losses in strength and mobility. When these go, everything we do, every move we make, requires a relatively higher percentage of our capacities thereby increasing injury risk. Our movements become less efficient, less stable, and less safe.

To be fragile: who would want *that*? I can't imagine why anyone would choose to be physically fragile. However, that is precisely, albeit by default, what folks are choosing when they forgo and miss out on strength training. The average baby boomer is, unfortunately, pretty darn fragile.

That's the bad news.

Bret Contreras, PhD, National Strength & Conditioning Association's current Personal Training Advisory Board representative posted something once that has become very popular throughout our industry: "If you think lifting weights is dangerous, try being weak. Being weak is dangerous."

The body, being the miracle that it is, responds to challenges to our current strength by adapting and getting stronger at virtually *any age*. Likewise, it can become more supple and more flexible. It can "learn to move well." Of the roughly forty-nine million sedentary baby boomers, how many have just resigned themselves to growing weaker, stiffer, and more fragile with a growing list of maladies, because they are intimidated and lack confidence and sufficient knowledge?

The strength gains I've been privileged to help my clients attain would amaze you. It amazed them! Yet they are no different from you. The strength training we do is often the first they've ever done. Here they are, taking it up in their fifties, sixties and some in their seventies. They say there are two best times to plant a tree: twenty years ago and right now, today. The same is true for starting a program of strength training. It's never too late. And, I promise you, you are far more capable than you imagine.

That's the good news.

Strength training is the single most important fitness endeavor, especially for our aging population. So, I'll try my best here to make it less intimidating and more easily understood, so you can undertake it with confidence.

Whether it's fat loss, firming, "toning," conditioning for an activity, metabolic health (think diabetes), or stability/balance to avoid falls, strength is the foundation for any goal we may have in mind.

###

Mobility. As children we had freedom of movement, unrestricted by fear of injury, and uncompromised by years of sitting, by that "premature rigor mortis" I mentioned earlier. One of my biggest influencers, Michael Boyle of Mike Boyle Strength & Conditioning, put it rather eloquently a while back with a "filet mignon versus beef jerky" analogy. As we get older our soft tissue—muscles, tendons, fascia—all degrade from a supple, filet mignon quality to one of a dry, brittle beef jerky-like quality. Through various methods we can restore some of that filet mignon quality. Mobility allows us to produce force, i.e., use our strength more efficiently, more safely.

Experts all over the Internet debate the effectiveness of stretching. It's been part of my personal fitness program for going on forty-five years now. I'm convinced the single biggest reason folks don't think its effective is because it's not being done while eliciting the relaxation response via conscious, diaphragmatic breath. Lack of patience and consistency are a couple other reasons.

Stretching alone probably isn't the best way to improve mobility but it can contribute. There are also those rare individuals for whom additional mobility is the last thing they need. So, indiscriminate stretching is a valid criticism. Mobility is distinct from, and more complex than, mere flexibility. Flexibility is the capacity of a muscle to stretch. Mobility refers to multiple factors affecting the function of, and movement at, a joint. I am confident the combined use of yoga poses, static stretches, dynamic stretching, and mobility drills (essentially stretching that involves movement) will help us improve mobility.

Another practice for improving mobility that's frequently debated, though more often about *how* it works than *if* it works, is foam rolling. Known as a self-myofascial release technique, it's also been called a "poor man's massage." You'll want to learn how to roll your upper back, your glutes/butt muscles, calves, inner thighs, and maybe quadriceps and hamstrings, too. And, you're gonna want to buy a foam roller for your home, so you can get that cheap massage between visits to the gym!

Improving strength, especially core (muscles that stabilize the spine) strength, can also help improve mobility. Generally speaking, as we gain strength and mobility, we become more stable, as well. When strength coaches discuss stability, they'll often declare, "You can't fire a cannon from a canoe!" One cannot produce efficient force and locomotion if one can't stabilize.

The ability to stabilize means we are able to prevent unwanted movement that otherwise creates energy leaks. Speaking of stability, falls among the elderly are a leading cause of injury and death, according to the CDC. And of those falls that are survived, unfortunately, they often mean the end of one's independence.

The effects of gravity—too much sitting and years of inactivity—create some "usual suspects." Everyone is different, but typically we'll need to address mobility in the shoulders, thoracic spine (upper back; both in extension and rotation), the hips, ankles, and even our feet.

I've used a simple, perhaps simplistic, analogy that seems to get the point across: mobility at joints is a bit like the alignment of your car's front end—when it's not right, the tires wear down prematurely, and the car doesn't roll as smoothly or efficiently. If we don't move efficiently at a given joint, not only is that joint affected, but there are often adverse effects that ripple up and/or down the body to other joints.

###

STRENGTH TRAINING PRINCIPLES #1 & # 2:

OVERLOAD & PROGRESSIVE OVERLOAD

THIS IS WHAT ALL that self-awareness, mindfulness, attachment/aversion, and addiction talk was intended to help you with. Effort, discomfort, exertion—they're all part of applying these two most important principles.

To make strength training effective, it must be a challenge to our current ability. This happens during a set (i.e., a given number of repetitions; lifting and lowering the weight start to finish), when we begin to exert a level of effort greater than we are accustomed.

Pay attention! This is important! Without this understanding and without the proper mindset, what usually happens is something I see all too often. A new client will be performing a lift. The first few repetitions are easy enough, but when it starts to get difficult, starts to feel a little uncomfortable, and starts to exceed their typical levels of exertion, they stop!

Without a mindful approach, as we start to encounter discomfort our thoughts tend to speed up, take on a frantic quality, and the mind protests. By the way, this is especially true in yoga. When we experience the inevitable discomfort of stiffness or of mobility restrictions in our body, the temptation to bail on a pose often wins out (remember Dr. Morita's quote). I tell my yoga students all the time, "A comfortable, tolerable discomfort is what we want."

I've joked with my training clients, suggesting the first several repetitions are just foreplay; the last two or three that we really work for are the main event. If we stop just as it begins to challenge us, we've essentially wasted our time. We are aiming to reach something close to a momentary muscle "failure," in which additional repetitions in good form become impossible without some rest.

We are trying to avoid momentary *mental* failure. The mind wants to give up well before our body's ability gives out. There is the now familiar notion, which has achieved cliché status, that the only growth that occurs does so outside our comfort zone. The key to success is to change our perspective on and our response to discomfort. We do that—you guessed it—by guarding our thoughts, inhabiting our body, and attending to our breath.

Progressive Overload is essentially the application of the Overload principle over time. As the body adapts and we get stronger, we will need to increase the stimulus in order to continue making progress. I think it's important to note, as we begin strength training, this will need to be done quite regularly, as strength increases occur quickly. It's not linear, however, and, over time, gains will slow down and level off.

George Leonard, in his little gem titled *Mastery,* talks about "loving the plateau," the maintenance between spikes of improvement. So, as long as we consistently apply the overload principle, we will maintain strength, continue to reap the benefits, and, on occasion, experience growth and improvement.

Overload can be accomplished in other ways besides just an increase in weight. For example, one can increase the volume of work (i.e., number of sets, reps, or exercises) or reduce the rest between exercises.

###

SOME VERY BASIC PROGRAM DESIGN PRINCIPLES

PERHAPS THE MOST IMPORTANT thing I can tell you about programs is there is no perfect program, there is no best program. One of the biggest challenges for someone new to strength training is where to begin, how to begin. This is make-or-break time. This is when most gym newbies wash out. The majority of new members, whether they join in January or July, don't last six months. So much can go wrong and too often does, in the first few weeks.

Most clubs offer an orientation/initial assessment as part of the membership. Our club does this, yet it is remarkable how many don't take us up on it. A truly thorough assessment, including a movement screen, is often beyond the skill set of the average trainer.

Finding a good trainer is not easy in this virtually unregulated industry. It may sound self-serving, but a competent one is worth his or her weight in gold. Often enough, folks need to be referred out to a qualified clinician, a physical therapist, or a physician well-versed in strength and conditioning. Most of us "of a certain age" will have injuries, conditions, etc. that must be accounted for when beginning and designing a workout program. This is my disclaimer, of sorts.

###

PLANES & PATTERNS

ALL OF US UNDERSTAND life in the physical world is a three-dimensional experience. But many of us don't appreciate how that relates to exercise.

Movement occurs in three planes: sagittal, frontal and transverse. Typical programs are heavy in only one, the sagittal. Google "planes of movement" and you can see an image depicting them. Just the act of walking involves movement and/or stabilizing in all three.

When our industry talks about functional training, I'd like to think this is one of the tenets it has in mind. Another is the concept of bodyweight mastery. A solid program will include strength and mobility work in all three planes of movement.

"Learn the rules like a pro, so you can break them like an artist."

—Pablo Picasso

When it comes to specific program design, to say there are an infinite number of possibilities is only a mild exaggeration. With all the variables that can be manipulated, there are endless options. Until recently, many if not most every program was some adaptation of bodybuilders' routines and involved a great deal of isolating muscle groups.

To go into any great detail regarding programming is beyond the scope of this "non-fitness" book. So, instead, I offer some general thoughts. With an understanding that the body functions as a unit and moves in multiple planes, programming for strength has shifted from body parts to movement patterns. These aren't the Ten Commandments; they aren't written in stone.

There are a few different takes on the concept of primary movement patterns. That said, this is what I use to program.

For the lower body:

> ➤ Hip Dominant (most of the movement occurs at the hip joint)
> ➤ Knee Dominant (knees bend and straighten more than in a hip dominant movement)

Both single leg (unilateral) and two leg (bilateral) should be programmed for both hip and knee dominant exercises.

For the upper body:

> ➤ Horizontal Pulling

- ➢ Vertical Pulling
- ➢ Horizontal Pushing
- ➢ Vertical Pushing

For the core/spinal stability:

- ➢ Anti-Extension & Anti-Rotation

And for the entire body:

- ➢ -Loaded Locomotion (e.g., farmer's carries)

These are the basics. There are additional components to a good, general program approach, but this is a good place to start.

###

GET HIP TO THE HINGE

ONE OF THE VERY FIRST things I go to work on with my clients is the ability to perform a hip hinge. This is money. Learning to keep the lumbar spine in neutral, to prevent it from rounding and keep it from becoming the loaded fulcrum when bending, is one of the keys to reducing the stress and strain to the lower back.

Too many of us have no idea how to "load the backside" to use the glutes (gluteus maximus/butt muscles) in order to spare the back and simultaneously engage the body's most powerful muscles in the most highly leveraged move the body is capable of performing.

[195]

The ill effects of sitting too much can create a movement deficiency that robs us of this ability and instead forces us to flex and load the lower back and overuse the quadriceps (front thigh muscles) and "abuse" the knees. Think about how many times in a given day you bend over, to take something out of the fridge or a low cabinet, picking things off the floor, and on and on. If, every time you bend, you do so poorly, just think of all the accumulated strain you've subjected the musculature, discs, and fascia of your lower back to, as well as your knees. Is it any wonder low back and knee pain (can you say patellofemoral pain syndrome?) are as common as they are among the aging population? How many times have we heard variations on the theme of the old, "I just bent over to pick up a pencil" scenario? (This postulation isn't without controversy, I readily acknowledge.)

Trust me, no product that a celebrity or athlete might hawk on TV is going to be nearly as effective in dealing with pain as the combination of mindfulness and quality movement. I implore my clients, after they learn to perform a hip hinge, to then program it into their bio-computer's (their brain's) software and use it throughout the day, every day, so it becomes automatic. If it becomes a "habit" in activities of daily living, it will be second nature in the gym.

This is why, after they learn the hip hinge, we start deadlifting, unless there's a compelling reason they shouldn't. The majority of my fifty-five-plus-year-old clients have ended up able to safely and easily lift his/her bodyweight in the deadlift.

None of this is to "fearmonger" and suggest your spine is going to explode, if you flex either your upper (thoracic) or lower (lumbar) spine, but learning and incorporating this move will serve you well.

The hip hinge is the King/Queen of movement skills.

###

RAGE AGAINST THE MACHINES... SORT OF

THERE ARE TWO COMMON scenarios. One is when the member will ask a trainer to show him or her how to use the machines. Chances are they've heard or otherwise believe machines to be safer than free weights. The other is when the orientation is little more than showing someone how to use the machines. Whichever the case, I feel the member is either doing, or being done, a disservice.

I ask folks to think about it this way: if your strength training routine consists entirely of going from one seated exercise machine to another seated exercise machine, all of which are performed in one plane of motion (the hip abduction/adduction machine being the only likely exception), where virtually all demands for stability, balance, and proprioception have been eliminated, then are we really getting the most from our time and effort? More than any other demographic, boomers need to be confident and stable on their feet. They stand to lose the most if and when they fall. Our time would be much better spent learning to move better. Recent research *has shown* machine training to offer more functional, transferable strength than previously thought or assumed. So, it doesn't have to be, nor should it be, an either-or proposition.

Nick Tumminello, another one of our industry's most brilliant minds, has convinced me to soften my militant stance against machines. He has distinguished himself as a champion of critical thinking, a challenger of "sacred cows," and one who coaxes the wild pendulum swings of popular sentiment back to a more moderate middle ground. Two of those pendulum swings have been the demonizing of machines and the dismissing of isolation exercises. Nick's dispassionate use of research and reason has done much to up the professionalism and down the dogma in this field.

Dan Ritchie, PhD and Cody Sipes, PhD, co-founders of the Functional Aging Institute, suggest in their book, *Never Grow Old*, that exercises be considered relative to where they might fall on a "functional continuum." I believe, for the vast majority of folks, especially us baby boomers, it's critical we expand our repertoire beyond the machines. My aim is to get clients to see the value of bodyweight mastery and to make that a priority.

The beauty of having a repertoire of bodyweight exercises is your "equipment" goes with you everywhere. I also want to show them how they can use resistance bands, free weights (e.g., kettlebells, dumbbells), medicine balls, and sandbags—tools that are inexpensive and take up little space. This approach also makes supplementing one's training in alternate settings outside the gym easier and far more likely.

###

STEVEN HEAD

SETS & REPS

SETS (A SUCCESSION OF reps, start to finish) and reps (short for repetitions) are the basic components of a strength exercise.

Prior to this book, the longest thing I'd ever written was a thirteen-page paper for clients and prospective clients entitled, *Fitness and You—Getting Started: A Practical and Philosophical Discussion.* I wrote it twenty-five years ago, and I still have one hard copy of it. It held up pretty well. The content, that is. In it, I discussed factors to consider when deciding how many reps one should perform. I suggested the specific number of reps performed in a set is not nearly as important as how challenging the last couple performed are. (It's all about that principle of overload.) If you want to do high reps with a comparatively lighter weight, you can still gain strength *if* you are working hard on the last couple reps. Recent research supports this. Studies have shown strength gains are possible by training up and down the rep range, using heavy weights that allow only a few reps, as well as lighter weights that can be done for higher reps.

As you gain strength in a given lift at a particular weight, the number of reps you can perform will increase. When you are consistently banging out ten or more reps at a given weight, that's the time to think about increasing the load. When you do, the reps you can now perform will decrease. A general guideline for increases is five to ten percent.

So, how many reps? There is no best answer. It depends on some rather specific training objectives, but, for general health benefits, it makes sense to mix it up. Just don't end your sets with any more than one or two reps left in the tank. Most of my clients do deadlifts, and we keep the reps between three and eight. Most of them do pushups as well (modified or otherwise), and reps can go as high as twenty-five.

One of the most enduring myths or fallacies is the notion that "high reps with low weights" is the key to toning and, if the goal is to put on muscle, to go with "heavier weight and lower reps." Not to be sexist, but this misconception often serves as an excuse for many women to avoid training hard. Not only do they often choose a light weight and do high reps (which we'll define here as twelve or more), but they also avoid the overload, which is the most essential requirement to derive any benefit at all. "Toning" will not occur otherwise.

Adults over fifty have already lost significant muscle and strength and will continue to do so without intervention. Most of us are at a genetic disadvantage in the first place when it comes to building muscle. Women, even more so. It doesn't help when we have high-profile "celebrity trainers" advising women not to lift anything over three pounds. That's tantamount to malpractice—certainly irresponsible. A gallon of milk weighs eight pounds, for crying out loud!

Another mistake I've seen quite often is folks will get a specific number in their head and believe there's magic in it. They think they *must* to do X number of reps. Often what happens is they will "beg, borrow, and steal" to get to that number. If, for whatever reason, they are fatiguing early in the set, they will shorten the range of motion and/or compromise their form just to reach the number. Get in the habit of doing only good, solid reps. Terminate the set at what is referred to as "technical failure," i.e., the point at which you can no longer perform good, solid reps.

What about sets? Again, it depends on a number of factors and considerations. One set per exercise is infinitely better than none. Two is more than twice as good as one, and three sets is where we start to think about the law of diminishing returns.

These are general notions for novice, general population trainees.

###

CONSISTENCY & VARIETY

"A foolish consistency is the hobgoblin of little minds."
—Ralph Waldo Emerson

"No man ever steps into the same river twice, for it is not the same river and he is not the same man."

—Heraclitus

CONSISTENCY AND VARIETY: both are important. Balancing the two is part of the artistry. Early on in one's training, consistency, or more specifically routine, is essential. Too much variety is actually not a good thing. It takes time to learn and get proficient at what may become your core or foundational exercises, those that most likely will be part of your program for life.

I tell my yoga students, depending on who you ask, there are anywhere from eighty-four to 8400+ yoga poses, but a basic core of a dozen or so can keep you challenged for at least this lifetime. The same holds true for strength training. Don't fall prey to Emerson's hobgoblin, though. As I mentioned earlier, with the numerous training variables and a little creativity, we can easily avoid doing the exact same thing over and over.

"The root cause of boredom is to be found in the obsessive search for novelty. Satisfaction lies in mindful repetition, the discovery of endless richness in subtle variations on familiar themes."

—George Leonard, from the book, *Mastery*

Consistency, as in regularity of training, is also key in the early going to ensure results, and results are powerful motivators. When you've been training a couple years consistently, missing or taking off a couple weeks isn't nearly as critical as it is in the first six months. That said, missing a workout here and there is inevitable.

Perhaps the second most important thing I can tell you about program design is one (you and it) must be "flexible." Life happens; there are inevitable, unavoidable "curve balls" that it throws at you. Too much insistence on adhering to a ridged schedule is a recipe for failure. Again, commitment to the big picture, the long haul, will help you stay on your feet. You will falter on occasion. However, there's no need for self-recrimination. You just pick yourself back up and carry on.

With a foundation well established, variety can be pursued a little more. My own strength training (as distinct from other aspects of my training), which must prepare me for the demands of baseball, isn't all that extensive. I do many of the same exercises every week, yet I rarely do the same workout twice in the same week—*subtle variations on familiar themes.*

There's an analogy about the goal of digging a well to find water: better to dig one well 100 feet deep than to dig ten wells ten feet deep. Don't be a program hopper. Don't chase novelty.

###

ROUTINES & REPERTOIRES

AKIN TO THE CONCEPTS of consistency and variety, the idea of routines and repertoires can keep us on the road to fitness success.

At the outset, having a couple routines works fine: an A and a B, if you train twice per week. If you get to the gym three days a week, you can alternate A-B-A with B-A-B on a weekly basis. Just two exercises in each of the patterns is a sufficient repertoire to make this approach work. Over time, you can build your repertoire of exercises.

You'll want enough routine to create consistency, and a repertoire big enough to allow for variety. Then your workouts can become less routine and more intrinsically driven creations. Make sense?

With this approach, you're going to develop self-efficacy, self-determination. Your workouts cease to be a chore you perform reluctantly, perfunctorily, and instead they will be challenges you take on with enthusiasm and focus. Unreasonable expectations give way to rewarding experiences.

###

MORE POWER TO YA'

AS IMPORTANT AS STRENGTH training is for us boomers to ensure our independence and optimize our health, power training may be *as* important, possibly more so. Research has shown it may have a greater impact on the ability to perform ADLs (activities of daily living) as we advance in age and a bigger role in fall prevention. And yet, it is another commonly overlooked component of fitness programing.

Put simply, power is work (force times distance) divided by time. Our basic strength work is done slowly, but power training exercises are performed fast. When was the last time you saw someone old move quickly and powerfully?

The loss of strength (particularly the decrease in the muscle fiber type responsible for quick, powerful contractions) combined with deteriorating nervous system efficiency (nerve conduction velocity) is a one-two punch that robs us of the ability to move quickly and produce force rapidly. The good news is it can be trained safely, once a solid strength base has been developed, *and* it can be a lot of fun!

Jumping, hopping, bounding, tossing, and slamming medicine balls—my older clients find this stuff exhilarating and... yes, empowering. I've had clients in their sixties and seventies who hadn't jumped in forty years or so work their way up to box jumps. They found the experience to be a tremendous confidence booster.

I have a sixty-two-year-old housewife for a client who, when she started with me a few years back, hadn't ever done any serious weight training. Just this week, I watched her doing kettlebell swings (an awesome exercise for power and work capacity) and realized she performs them better than I do!

For some, power training might mean just pedaling an exercise bike at a challenging RPM for short intervals. For others it might be box jumps or swinging a twenty-kilo kettlebell.

The capacity to react and move quickly can help avoid or minimize an injury and perhaps even save your life in an emergency.

It's hard to move fast if you only train slow.

###

MINDSET MISSTEP #3

THE TIME WARP

"Those who cannot find time for recreation are obliged sooner or later to find time for illness."

—John Wanamaker

"You can pay me now, or you can pay me later."

—The auto mechanic in an old FRAM oil filter commercial

LACK OF TIME IS ONE of the biggest, most common excuses we have for not exercising. And one of the big misconceptions about exercise is that it takes a prohibitive investment in time to be of value.

When I went the through the local car wash recently, the manager looked at me and said, "Damn! You must live in the gym! Look at those forearms—those are baseball player forearms!" He had that much right. He proceeded to speculate how many days and how many hours I spent working out.

I told him, "I work in the gym, but I don't live there." Even with the greater demands of training for a sport, I put in, on average, three to four sessions per week, ranging anywhere from thirty to seventy-five minutes long. That's hardly "living" at the gym.

Quality time. When it comes to exercise, more is not necessarily better. Smarter and more efficient is better. Generally speaking, intensity is more important than duration. The big exception is, of course, endurance-event goals.

Intensity and duration are inversely related. The more intense our training, the shorter in duration it must be. That comes as great news for folks who thought they had to toil for an hour on the treadmill or lift weights for hours at a time. Every day, I see folks sitting on the bikes, pedaling for extended periods of time with hardly any effort or intensity, just logging their time, when they could be achieving far greater benefit in far less time. More on this in a bit.

Food diaries are often used to help folks become more aware of what and how much they actually eat. A time diary could do the same regarding how we actually spend our time. No doubt many of us piss away a fair amount of time. That said, it's not mere semantics to say we need to make the time as opposed to find it.

###

PAIN & ABLE

"In the soil of the quick fix is the seed of a new problem, because our quiet wisdom is unavailable."

—Wayne Muller

IN HIS BOOK, *A Guide to Better Movement,* Todd Hargrove opens the chapter entitled, "The Science of Pain" with a quote by noted neuroscientist, Vilayanur Ramachandran: "Pain is an opinion."

The chapter is a fascinating read on the complexities of pain, our experience of it, and all the various factors that influence it.

This is one of my soapbox issues: how so many of us deal with pain. Pain may be an opinion of sorts; it most certainly should be an invitation, an opportunity. There is much to learn from pain, if we are willing to listen, give it some space, and not fight it so much.

Instead, we are a culture that seems determined to ignore most of what we might learn about the incredible body we inhabit, in order to dull or kill the pain. We want a quick fix. We don't seem interested in that "quiet wisdom." Often that quick fix lands us in a real fix—too quick to assume our doctor is acting in our best interest. Look at our nation's opioid crisis: killer painkillers.

To be clear, I am not unsympathetic. Nor am I suggesting we be irresponsible when medical attention is the prudent course of action. I've known pain that I felt I wouldn't survive without some pharmacological intervention. During the worst of my depression, I went through a stretch in which I did not attend to my oral health so well. I ended up with an abscess, the pain from which was so bad, if I had had a gun in the house, who knows.

I'm talking primarily chronic pain here: on and off again orthopedic "aches and pains."

"A little *bit of pain never hurt anybody."*

—Steven Head

We all have varying capacities for pain tolerance. I get it. What I also get is many of us are in far too big a hurry to run to the medicine cabinet or be talked into prescriptions or surgery in circumstances where we'd be much better off giving the body a chance to work together with time and intelligent movement. The mindfulness practice I've just spent several pages advocating for, in order to help us tolerate the discomfort associated with exercise, can be one of our best strategies in dealing with pain, as well.

"No man ever steps into the same river twice, for it is not the same river and he is not the same man."

—Heraclitus

See what I did there? When it comes to pain, our experience of it, the Heraclitus quote is worth repeating.

I mentioned the psychological term "premature cognitive commitment." For years, I've contended that the anticipation and fear of pain is often more debilitating than the pain itself. What do we typically do when we anticipate pain? We tighten up, stiffen, and hold our breath. Not the best strategy. The anticipation can, in fact, create a bit of a self-fulfilling prophecy. Just because an activity caused pain once does not necessarily mean it will the next time.

Diagnosis is *not* destiny. An unfavorable MRI should not be considered the final, definitive word. For some, this may be the single most important takeaway from this book.

Dr. James Andrews, one of the most highly regarded, widely respected sports medicine doctors and orthopedic surgeons once said, essentially (he specifically was referring to baseball players), if you want an excuse to perform surgery, you do an MRI. The point being people without pain or dysfunction will often have MRIs showing damage or abnormalities. Conversely, a fair number of folks will present with pain even in the absence of abnormal imaging. Pain and the diagnosing of injury, it seems, aren't as black and white as a black and white image might suggest.

Over the years, in my initial sessions with clients, I often ask them to ride the bike while I sit next to them. We chat. This is where I get a feel for their experiences, their history, their stories, and their mindset. Countless times, I've listened to accountings of what they've been told by their doctors they couldn't or shouldn't do anymore. I've listened to what they used to be able to do, yet are convinced they cannot anymore. I've had several tell me, "Oh, I can't ride the bike—it hurts my knees."

I will ask," Well, when was the last time you rode a bike?" (When did you last step into the river?)

"About ten years ago."

Pain is such a fluid, mercurial thing; our experience of it can change from day to day, hour to hour. I have learned so much just by giving space to the experience of pain. So have a number of my clients. The number of fairly significant pains I've experienced (in a hip, a knee, a shoulder, or the muscles of the mid-back) that arrived almost inexplicably and disappeared rather spontaneously a day or three later must number in the hundreds by now.

All without Advil or Aleve.

I'll share a personal anecdote, one of the most powerful ones, because it wasn't just a run-of-the-mill, chronic "aches and pains" scenario. This was an acute trauma situation.

I'd torn my left medial meniscus sliding during a ball game in 2002. That was the official diagnosis by a noted sports medicine orthopedist in my area. I went to see him about a week after the incident. I was hobbled, the pain and swelling so bad I could not bear weight on it. Classic symptoms. Confident diagnosis. He recommended I have surgery. I told him I already had backcountry passes and airline tickets for a climb of Mt. Whitney less than three weeks away. "When you get back, then."

After a little more than a week, I could tolerate some load bearing, so I began pulling up the carrots to see how they were growing. That's an analogy I use to describe the careful process of determining how the recovery is progressing: what hurts, what doesn't, and how much function has been regained.

The injury occurred on June 2. On June 19, I was standing on the summit of the highest mountain on the continental United States. I've gone on to play seven months of baseball every year since. The next year, 2003, I incurred the very same injury (though not from sliding) to my right medial meniscus. Same symptoms, same severity. Same outcome. No unnecessary surgery.

Diagnosis is *not* destiny.

"Movement hurts, but not moving destroys. Incorrect movement harms, but intelligent movement heals."

—Mary Pullig Schatz, M.D.

While I was writing this book, I conducted a number of informal surveys on Facebook, asking just one question: "If you do not currently exercise, what is your primary reason/excuse?"

Each was a small sample size, but most of those who responded were actually baby boomers. The most common reasons cited for not exercising were injuries (often old injuries) and chronic pain.

This was disheartening to hear. The body is an amazing thing—a marvel of regenerative capacities. It's capable of alchemy, whereby it can take a positive mindset, mix it with intelligent movement, and often yield "medicine."

###

SUCCESS STRATEGY # 1

VERSUS

MINDSET MISSTEP #3

SOMEWHERE EARLY ON in my training, I realized I would often try to convince myself I was too tired to work out. I probably succeeded in doing so a time or two. But, like allowing just one weed in your garden, you soon find it's overrun with them.

I couldn't keep doing that and keep up my consistency. I decided to question, to challenge that voice in my head. I decided to "sign a contract" with myself. I promised myself, whenever I had thoughts of being too tired, I would get to the gym (for years, I kept a membership at a gym other than where I worked) and start the workout, usually with some cardio (e.g., bike, stair climber). If, after ten minutes, I still felt too tired to work out, if it felt wrong, like I really *shouldn't* exercise, then I would abort the mission.

I've employed this strategy for decades. In all that time, in the hundreds and hundreds of times I felt "too tired," I think I've walked out on the workout less than a handful of occasions. In fact, I've gone on to have some of my best workouts after having thought I was too tired.

I've also allowed myself the flexibility, given myself permission, to abridge the workout and do less than I had originally planned, when I thought it prudent. This, and a commitment to getting the session started, will help you avoid the all-or-none trap.

[229]

- ➤ Mental fatigue.
- ➤ Aversion to effort.
- ➤ Desire for comfort.

These are what conspire to convince you to blow off the workout. They are a very persuasive triumvirate. If you still work for a living, you probably know that feeling at the end of the day: you just want to go home and plop on the couch (a big reason many folks train in the morning before work).

The fatigue you feel is almost certainly mental—a product of stress and inactivity. Movement, which increases blood flow, does an amazing job of burning off the fog of mental fatigue. I can't tell you how many times I've had clients show up for their session tired and uninspired, only to get through it with some music and a little humor. At the end of our session, they'll look at me and say, "I feel less tired now than when I got here. I feel better now than before the workout."

That's when I will say, "Remember this—this is huge! Next time you're tempted to cancel or blow off a workout on your own, because you think you're too tired, remember how the workout actually *gave* you energy."

Numerous times, I've said to folks, if you feel like you need a nap but can't get one, a short, light workout is easily the next best thing. Yes, there have been and will be occasions when you just know you shouldn't exercise, but they are rare, in comparison. Greater self-awareness (mind and body) will help us distinguish between the two and keep the weeds from winning out.

Honor the contract. Keep that promise.

###

SUCCESS STRATEGY # 2:

DETAIL THE SWEATS

THERE'S SOMETHING REALLY gratifying about documenting one's workouts. When I first started lifting weights, I kept a training log. At that time, it was to be able to track progress, to analyze the effectiveness of my training. But, at the time, it wasn't really a source of gratification.

I kept a log until the early eighties before giving it up. In November 2014, I decided to begin keeping a training log again. I bought one of those nice, hardbound journals with the blank pages. I had a sense this was a record I was going to want to have when the time came to up my visibility in, and my impact on, this field. Not sure exactly to what end. Time will tell.

I don't carry the log/journal around during the workout, like I did back in the day. Rather, I log every exercise, every set, and each rep in my head. When I get home, I eagerly and with great satisfaction write down the workout. These days, keeping a log is *very* gratifying.

Doing so will go a long way to help you hone your instincts and increase your familiarity with program elements. It can help keep you on track and motivated.

###

SUCCESS STRATEGY #3:

THE BUDDY SYSTEM

"As iron sharpens iron, so one man sharpens another."
—Proverbs 27:17

FINDING A FRIEND to work out with can be a very effective strategy, if you are both committed to keeping each other accountable.

For various reasons, I have trained by myself most of my life. But the times in which I've trained with a partner have been rewarding. I have a former client who has become a good friend, and we train together on occasion. It creates a dynamic that helps us dig a little deeper, as well as enjoy it a little more.

That said, we don't want a "blind leading the blind" scenario. This is where I make the case for hiring a trainer. For many, hiring a trainer for an extended period of time isn't feasible. But hiring a good one for even a couple weeks is an investment that will pay dividends for a very long time.

As a trainer, my job is to believe in my new client more than they believe in themselves. It's my job to push them a little harder than they'd push themselves— not to coddle them, but not to crush them, either. To meet them where they are. It is to help them overcome their own limiting beliefs, to address the misinformation, and to dispel the misconceptions they come to me with.

A good trainer provides both what the client wants and what the client needs but does so in a manner that's consistent with their goals and does no harm.

The key is to program in such a way that achieves those aims but also gets buy-in from the client.

Primum non nocere.

Of the countless number of folks who set New Year's fitness resolutions only to wash out before Valentine's Day, I wonder how many would have survived, even thrived, had they only hired a knowledgeable coach for a time.

Tribe. Community. I hear these terms used to describe the camaraderie many people experience when they join a club, or, more to the point, what keeps them coming back. The social component, this connection, should not be underestimated. It has worked well for others; it could work for you.

###

CARDIO OR WEIGHTS? YES, BUT...

I REMEMBER WHEN CARDIO (short for cardiovascular or cardio-respiratory) was crowned king. The aerobics revolution began with Dr. Kenneth Cooper's work in the late sixties and early seventies. He put jogging on the map.

To this day, the notion that running/jogging or aerobics in general is the best, smartest way to lose weight and get fit endures. Many folks today still embark on their quest for fitness by taking up jogging and don't even consider strength training. For years, cardio was cardio and weights were weights, and never the twain would meet. With what we now know about energy systems and metabolic responses, it seems the twain have, in fact, met.

I was talking with a prospective client recently who stated his primary goal was weight loss, and he immediately declared, "But I hate running."

I told him, "Well, you're in luck." He, too, was under the impression that running was the activity of choice for weight loss.

Running isn't only unnecessary, it can be a poor choice in the long run, especially for us older folks. Many don't tolerate it well orthopedically; it isn't particularly friendly to joints. Those who are vulnerable to "boredom" often find it mind-numbing.

Running and strength training are in effect at odds with one another in that they are "competing" for the body's limited capacity to respond and adapt. As mentioned earlier, us baby boomers are already behind the eight-ball when it comes to preserving strength. In an effort to become more efficient at running, the body will give up muscle, which is counterproductive.

Muscle is like the engine of a car: it burns fuel and makes us go. Continuing the analogy, it is what determines the idle speed, i.e., how much energy the car is using at rest. The number of calories burned in a given workout is only half the story. Strength training, particularly certain formats, can rival cardio in terms of caloric expenditure during the session, but in addition will boost the body's idle in the hours after the workout and, over time, create a higher, more active metabolism.

LSD, as it's been called—long slow distance; low intensity, steady-state cardio—does not do that for us. Muscle is highly active, metabolically. It requires energy to maintain. So, the more muscle we have (and I don't mean in aggregate, but as a percentage of bodyweight), the more calories we burn while watching TV, driving, and even sleeping. Muscle is good. Muscle is your friend!

So, getting back to the cardio/weight intersection. The aerobic (meaning with oxygen) energy system in our body is always on. It is the primary source of energy, unless and until we step up the intensity of activity. For that, we have two other energy systems that provide fuel when the aerobic system can't meet the demands. They are referred to as anaerobic (without oxygen). Activities that cause us to breathe heavily—e.g., a run up some stairs, set of squat jumps, or a set of kettlebell swings—require big contributions from these anaerobic energy systems.

String enough of these together and the aerobic capacity (one of the primary aims of cardio) gets developed as well. Combine two to four strength training exercises in rapid succession and do that multiple times in a workout: the same thing. So, we can get comparable as well as additional benefits in less time, typically, without the drawbacks.

Yes to cardio? Yes, but in moderation and not to the exclusion of strength training, more as a lower priority. And, like the machines versus free-weight debate, it shouldn't be an either/or proposition. It just behooves us to have a better understanding of how they all relate. I still do some steady-state cardio, but as a supplement to my strength training and almost never more than twenty minutes.

Even the traditional cardio activities like elliptical trainers, exercise bikes, stair climbers, and treadmills can be made more efficient, both metabolically and time wise, if we are willing to work a bit harder at them. Instead of comparatively low effort, steady-state approach, one can regularly (not necessarily every time) do intervals, whereby short duration, high effort bouts are alternated with a longer, low-effort recovery intervals and then repeated.

A typical starting point is the two-to-one rest:work

ratio. Using the exercise bike as an example, it might look something like this: the work interval for thirty seconds at ninety to a hundred RPMs (pedal rate) at Level 8, then the rest interval for sixty seconds of sixty to seventy RPMS at Level 2.

The term "cardio" is slowing giving way to "energy system development" and "conditioning," both suggesting that "cardio" is a bit more complex than generally understood. This is especially true for those who train athletes. How the body adapts to a given stimulus is highly specific, so training should reflect that.

I won't go into it much beyond this, but it's a fundamental exercise physiology principle, known as the S.A.I.D. principle: Specific Adaptation to Imposed Demands. I train a number of recreational tennis and baseball players. In addition to the concept of power training coming as a surprise, they are often unaware that the steady-state cardio they do for their training probably isn't the best choice for their sport's demand.

For those of us who want to exercise for "general health," to improve our ability to function in daily activities, lower our risk of injury and disease, and enhance our efforts to engage in life as a verb, we'll want to develop an overall work capacity that is a combination of both strength and aerobic endurance.

###

STEVEN HEAD

SUZIE STAIRMASTER
SYNDROME
A Cautionary Tale

THIS IS A (TRUE) STORY I've recounted numerous times as a teaching moment, about the importance of good form, dilution of effort, and deluding of self.

In 1989, I worked at a club where we had a couple first-generation StairMasters, the 4000PT, with independently moving pedals and about fifteen inches of travel that simulated climbing stairs. It had handrails, and the computer console graphics consisted of columns and rows of red dots. The height of the columns denoted the speed/difficulty setting, and the column itself, an interval of time. At the end of a workout, they would be displayed across the width of the screen.

A young woman came in almost every day to work out on one of them. Invariably (the machine was situated right next to a main walkway, so it was easy to see this), she would use it on the manual setting and crank the speed as high as it would go, represented by a column of the red dots that went from the bottom of the display screen to the top. She would set the interval time so the workout was an hour long. When she finished, the display was completely covered with red lights.

You'd be tempted to think, wow, that's some amazing aerobic endurance to be able to climb stairs at the fastest setting for an hour. And all those calories burned! She probably thought the same thing, herself. At the end of the workout, the screen would read out the estimated calories.

But, what the machine didn't know was she placed her hands on the rails, fingers pointing back toward her, and pushed into the rails, displacing her body weight, lifting a large percentage of it off the pedals, and then "fluttered" them through about a three- or four-inch range of motion for the duration of the workout. She had effectively reduced the workload by probably sixty percent or more with this "technique." So, when the machine told her she'd burned 450 calories (a rough estimate in the first place), the reality is she hadn't burned anything close to that.

I can only surmise, but it's a pretty safe bet she was stroking her ego and, in the process, deluding herself about what incredible shape she was in and how many calories she'd actually burned.

The story of Suzie StairMaster doesn't end there. She was conspicuous in a weeklong absence, and when she returned, she had a brace on both wrists. Suzie had developed carpel tunnel syndrome as a result of all the stress she'd subjected her wrists to by her cheating the machine.

Though not to this extreme, I still see folks doing this on our stair climbers. It's not uncommon to see people crank the incline way up on the treadmills, ostensibly to work harder and burn more calories, but then lean back with arms extended and hold on. They end up in the same gait pattern and body position they'd be with the treadmill level but with no natural arm swing. That wouldn't be possible walking up an actual hill/incline. And they negate most any increase in intensity they sought to effectuate.

Form matters. Technique has consequences. Better to check the ego, dial back the workload (the weight, if lifting), and perform the activity with good form.

"Learning is the very essence of humility, learning from everything and everybody. There is no hierarchy in learning."

—Krishnamurti

This is another argument for getting with a good trainer. Every day, I see examples of training that suggests an absence of basic knowledge. Most of us didn't study kinesiology or biomechanics or exercise physiology in school. It stands to reason, if we didn't, there may be much we don't know that we don't know, when it comes to effective exercise.

Too many of us live in a body we know very little about. The best athletes in the world have coaches. Don't be that guy who says to me after I offer to lend a professional perspective, "I played football in high school. I'm good."

###

BRINGING MR. DUFFY HOME

"Attention or conscious concentration on almost any part of the body produces some direct physical effect on it."

—Charles Darwin

"He who feels it, knows it more."

—Bob Marley

I HAD AN AHA MOMENT this weekend while at a conference.

One of the presenters mentioned the concept of the "mind-muscle connection." I probably first heard of it thirty-five-plus years ago, during my bodybuilding "phase." Put simply, during a strength training exercise, focusing intently on the muscles involved and paying close attention to the sensations, the experience of the effort can actually enhance the body's response to it.

Many of us have not been very good to our bodies. And, conversely (chicken or egg), our bodies have not been very good to us. Either one suggests we are likely "deficient" in body awareness. This lack of body awareness has been very apparent over the years, as I've trained adults who are new to exercise.

Some of us are going to struggle with adhering to a formal meditation practice, especially in the early going. Hell, I'm still challenged to be consistent. What can help tremendously, either as an alternative or as a complementary practice, is the *body scan*.

In addition to formal meditation and yoga, the body scan is an integral part of Dr. Kabot-Zinn's program at UMass. The body scan is essentially a mental tour of the body, to shine a spotlight of awareness on physical sensations, one body part or region at a time. It can be done lying down. It's a powerful tool for developing greater body awareness, which can be effective in ameliorating chronic pain, which I alluded to earlier.

And using the scan will improve our mind-muscle connection, which can transform the discomfort of exercise exertion from something intolerable to something quite incredible, not to mention help kick boredom in the ass! If you search YouTube for "guided body scan meditation," you'll find videos of various lengths, from five minutes to an hour or more.

###

DO NOT GO GENTLE

IT'S NEVER TOO LATE. Until, it is.

For many of you who are members of this book's intended audience, it's not. Not yet. If you're still able to walk and to get up out of a chair, count your blessings.

I know life hasn't been as kind to some as it has to others. But most of us who aren't doing anything can do something. And the incredible thing is many of us are sitting on a gold mine of potential. You have no idea how incredibly fit, strong, active, healthy, and pain free you could become, if you just made that decision to embark on the journey.

The stories are out there, lots of them, of people who hadn't exercised most or all of their adult life and who have gone on to run obstacle course races, compete in masters competitions in various sports, or "just" see a whole new world of activity and adventure open up for them.

The first part of this book, the memoir part, I shared my story with you, to connect and hopefully inspire. It was to show how I arrived here, sixty-one years into a life, more than half of which has been spent in this profession, and from whence comes my passion and my motivation.

This second part, the "manual" portion, is offered up to help you navigate the psychological mine field, as I have come to recognize it, and to share some basic (very basic) training knowledge in the hopes of making the first few steps of your journey easier, to give you a better chance of success, and maybe help you better vet a prospective trainer.

With apologies to Dylan Thomas:

Do not go gentle into that good night.
Old age should yearn to move until the close of day.
Train and rage against the dying of your might.

Mindset Matters Most. That's the title of a short but profound book written by the author of this book's foreword, Brian Grasso. One of the foundational tenets in his work worldwide, as a business and life coach, is that to achieve success in any facet of life in which it's eluded you thus far is not necessarily to learn more strategies for that success, but rather to get conscious to and eliminate the reasons why it's eluded you in the first place.

Learn how and why you are in your own way.

Having someone in your corner, someone who believes in you, can go a long way in helping you achieve success. I'm already there.

[254]

In closing, I want to leave you with a couple stories. They speak to two of the most important messages I hope to convey. I want to express my deep, heartfelt thanks for taking the time to read my book.

Peace and Love.

Let's connect!

I invite you and other readers to meet up with me on the Facebook page for *Not Another Fitness Book:*

www.facebook.com/NotAnotherFitnessBook

My personal Facebook page is:

www.facebook.com/Steven.Head.984

If you are interested in exploring online or distance coaching, feel free to email me here:

steven@headstrong.fitness

STEVEN HEAD

THE STOLEN AXE
(Courtesy of Tao-how.blogspot.com)

ONE COLD MORNING, a farmer went out to chop wood and realized his axe was missing. He always kept the axe in the same place, next to the woodpile. Now, it was nowhere to be seen.

"I'll bet that boy next door took it," he thought. "That kid's always watching me. And he's so quiet. He seems like the sneaky type who would steal something. I'll keep an eye on him…"

The next day, the man watched the young boy whenever he was outside. The boy seemed nervous and jumpy. "He's guilty as sin," thought the man. "I bet he knows I'm on to him. Look at the way he walks, with his head down, like he's ashamed of something."

Later that evening, the farmer decided to go into town and purchase a new axe. "But I'll keep an eye on that kid for a few days," he thought. "He'll slip up soon enough, and when he does, I'll catch him!"

The man walked out to the barn to saddle up his horse, and when he did, he saw the axe. There it was, just inside the door. He had brought it in for sharpening two days ago and completely forgotten about it.

The next morning, the man saw the boy out in the yard again. The boy was doing the same things he had always done—walking around, sitting on the steps, performing a few chores—but something was different about him.

"What a nice young man," thought the farmer. "He's so quiet and polite, spending time with his family and doing his chores every morning… "I was a fool to think someone like that could steal from me."

###

THE SECRET OF LIFE

I FOUND THIS STORY recounted in Kathleen A. Brehoney's *Awakening at Midlife*. She says it's one that is told in India concerning an argument among the gods on where to hide the secret of life, so humans will not find it.

"Bury it under a mountain," one god suggested. "They'll never find it there."

"No," the others countered. "One day, they will find a way to dig up the mountain and uncover the secret of life."

STEVEN HEAD

"Put it in the depths of the deepest ocean," another god suggested. "It will be safe there."

"No," said the others. "Someday, humankind will find a way to travel to the depths of the ocean and will find it."

"Put it inside them," another god said. "Men and women will never think of looking for it there."

All the gods agreed, and so it is said the gods hid the secret of life within us.

###

ACKNOWLEDGMENTS

I WISH TO EXPRESS special thanks to a few folks, without whom this book would never have been written. They are: Brian Grasso, Carrie Campbell, AJ Mihrzad, Pat Pilla, Andrew Friedman, Dallas Hudgens.

To a few others who have been highly influential professionally, to whom I also owe a debt of gratitude. They are: Michael Boyle, Eric Cressey, Mark Verstegen, Nick Tumminello, Brett Jones, Gray Cook, Tony Gentilcore, Betsey Downing, PhD, Bret Contreras, PhD, Martin Rooney, Joe Sansalone, Karen McDowell Smith, Darius Andre Gilbert.

To the countless clients in the past thirty-five years with whom I've had the privilege of working, notably four in particular whose support has spanned more than a decade. They are Jeff & Anne Martin, and Mike & Suha Atassi.

To the neighborhood gang—"Whit," "Wilkie," "Cog," Curt & "Sutt."

To Dad, Colonel Willie C. "Chet" Head, Jr. & Mom, Ardella Helen Head.

And lastly, to a woman who showed me I was, in fact, loveable. Thank you, Alicia.

###

ABOUT THE AUTHOR

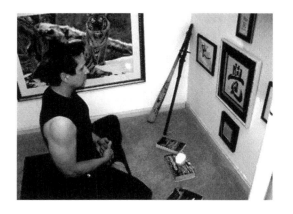

STEVEN HEAD, CSCS is a personal trainer, strength coach, and yoga teacher in McLean, Virginia. Steven's career in fitness spans five decades. He has worked independently and in physical therapy clinics, large health clubs, and small "boutique shops." He has worked with teens, septuagenarians, and everyone in between.

His clients have included heads of state, members of Congress, business CEOs, and elite athletes, but mostly just ordinary folks hoping to find help in becoming healthier. When he isn't working with clients, he is practicing what he preaches or playing baseball, pool, reading, or enjoying the company of friends.

He lives in Herndon, Virginia.

###

Made in the USA
Lexington, KY
20 November 2019